ACTS of
KINDNESS

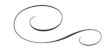

ACTS of KINDNESS

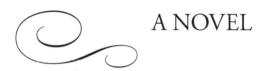

A NOVEL

by
Catherine A. Hosmer

iUniverse, Inc.
New York   Bloomington

ACTS OF KINDNESS

iUniverse books may be ordered through booksellers or by contacting:

iUniverse
1663 Liberty Drive
Bloomington, IN 47403
www.iuniverse.com
1-800-Authors (1-800-288-4677)

ISBN: 978-1-4401-1492-2 (pbk)
ISBN: 978-1-4401-1493-9 (ebk)

Printed in the United States of America

iUniverse rev. date: 02/18/2009

Acknowledgements

The author wishes to thank the following people for their help in producing this book:

Dr. Richard Redfern, professor emeritus of English, Clarion University of Pennsylvania, for his skillful editing of this manuscript

John A. Hosmer, M.D., my husband, now deceased, for his medical expertise while the manuscript was being written

Jerry D. Moore, M.D., retired general surgeon, for checking medical facts in the Chapter One operating scene

This book was inspired by an article, *Benign Violence*, written by Mark Kramer and appearing in *Atlantic Monthly*

CHAPTER ONE

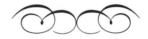

Bairstow knows what the trouble is even before he leaves home for the hospital this morning. He'd been reading the funnies in the *Boston Globe*, planning to transfer eventually to the book section of the *New York Times*, when the call came in. He'd even been expecting surgery this Sunday morning; after all, three of the last five mornings when he'd been on duty there'd been an emergency of some kind. He's even arranged his clothes so that he can snag them in a hurry, on the run: shirt, pants, sweater, to hell with the suit jacket; he'll save that for the office tomorrow. At least on Sunday, emergency day, all of that can be eliminated. He's even grown to like Sunday, when all the excess motion can be razed from his professional life, when the action becomes pure and simple allowing him to deal with life's emergencies and complications on a more rarified plane.

The trouble is that this patient knows precisely what is going on, but perhaps this is an asset, too, when one weighs the pros and cons of the procedure, as Bairstow is doing this minute, rapidly dressing, throwing on those clothes so carefully laid out for just such a moment as this. For the woman is a former nurse, now 58, whose medical knowledge just might, now that he thinks of it, have given her a chance of survival--not a good one, to be sure, but at least a chance. Ten years ago (Bairstow can pinpoint the time almost exactly because he himself was just entering practice and she was one of his first patients) she'd undergone a procedure at a New York hospital whereby a nylon artery had been installed in place of a damaged one in her malfunctioning heart. Maybe it had saved her life then, Bairstow thinks, buttoning the last button on his shirt and pulling the belt snugly about his waist, but it surely is killing her now because that nylon has eroded, as it so often does in those old procedures. No one used nylon anymore, and the nurse, Helen Proctor, had understood that, too. She's watched--no, monitored--herself for all those many years for signs of that critical deterioration, for that precise moment when the process would begin to leak, and this very morning she'd thought she detected it.

Bairstow's phone had rung minutes ago. "I feel it, Dr. Bairstow," she'd said, coolly, calmly. She'd never in her life called him Ben despite the easy familiarity between nurses and doctors, the dirty jokes and medical innuendoes, not only because she's a patient now, but for the additional reason that she's a formal, private woman. "There's something *there*, it feels like indigestion."

"You're sure it's not indigestion, Helen, not gallbladder, or..." Bairstow began to journey down the gamut of other things which might be guilty of the feeling of distress to his patient, but he stopped because Helen knows herself as few of his other patients do.

"No, it isn't. It feels as if...something's escaping, dripping away."

That's it, then, a circulatory system which just might be emptying itself...and they'd only know for sure when they went in to discover the source of the odd pain...well, not pain exactly, the discomfort that might be nothing...or might indicate seepage just below the fastening of the old nylon prosthesis to the stump of the aorta.

"Please go immediately to the hospital," Bairstow had said to the woman. I'll arrange everything. Do you have someone at home with you?"

"No. My cats only. I live alone. I'll drive myself in."

Bairstow had chewed his lip at that, it was almost frightening, but he understood the solitary fact: she'd not take an ambulance even if he ordered one, she'd drive herself. That much he understood, and he had to deal with that knowledge.

Hurriedly he'd called the hospital, talking to the emergency crews: the patient would be arriving, they were to watch for her, to monitor her immediately, they were to take her into their hallowed circles and minister unto her in the best, most rapid, most thorough way they could manage. She was one of their own, Bairstow implied as much, knowing he was acting in a dictatorial and high-handed way but not caring, implying that it would be on their heads if she were to die. He liked the patient particularly and admired her pluck and fortitude.

Then Bairstow called his partner, Jefferson Potter: he was off today, but had informed Bairstow that he'd be "around," which meant that he could be contacted. Bairstow knows little about Potter personally despite their close professional association of three years' duration; the two men live across town from each other, Potter is 35, 10 years younger than Bairstow. He trained in Philadelphia, he's somewhat introverted, has some kind of difficulty with his marriage, but Bairstow has never even met Potter's wife. That's the sum total of what he knows about Potter, except that Potter's a good surgeon though not awfully experienced. Beyond that Bairstow doesn't give a damn.

"Problem," Bairstow had informed Potter's surprisingly awake voice. "Helen Proctor. Sounds as if her prosthesis might be breaking down. I'll need you. Can you come?"

"Ten minutes," Potter answered. "No traffic cross-town. Hospital in a half-hour."

Normally Potter is a man of few words, and today especially so with the emergency. Today Bairstow is grateful: he's had his hands full. Besides, he's got to hurry to Memorial Hospital, too, now that he's allowed sufficient time for the troops to muster. He, too, can make it in 10 minutes without traffic. Usually the rituals of Bairstow's surgery begin a day ahead, and are as proscribed as if preparing for a space shot: bathing, medicines, purgatives, tests, visits by consultants, the laying-on of hands. Not today. Today everyone gets cast into the void of sudden jeopardy, of instant decision. Bairstow's hair on the back of his neck begins to prickle as it always does when he feels the tension of the case, like electricity in the air--but on occasion he hasn't denied to himself that he functions well, smoothly, with precision in the stir of events, the throb of adventure, the focus of attention. But the fact that he can help, that he might save a life, is out there, too.

Before he leaves home, the phone rings again: it's Peggy Hagerty, the emergency room nurse. "Your patient has arrived," she says. "She looks pale, pasty, shocky. Blood pressure 90 over 50. We're preping her..."

"Give me time, I'm coming..." How the hell did Helen get there so fast, Bairstow wonders, she must have driven on two wheels. Then he recalls that she lives on a street beside the hospital. Of course, he thinks, she's been waiting for this event for years, trying to anticipate this moment of disaster by moving near the hospital to give herself an edge on life.

Bairstow waves quickly to his wife, far back in the cave of his house, where she and the two kids still at home are cleaning up after breakfast: the oldest, a daughter, is in prep school. He can see his wife's face even from where he's standing in the front hall. She's wearing a bright apron and waves back. He comes and goes so often that for her there is no loss in it: he will return, and she goes about her business.

Bairstow climbs into his car: it's a Lexus, and he's just purchased it this spring. As Bairstow gazes across the hood, he can see dust: occasionally he's furtively taken his handkerchief and polished the slick surface until the offending blemish disappears and the shine returns. After all, his father was a poor man who owned seedy second-hand cars his entire life, and this luxury of possessing an expensive, well-honed machine satisfies some secret craving he hadn't even known he'd harbored in his heart-of-hearts until recently.

He backs from his circular drive, enters the lane of traffic and levels the nose of his car down the road, feeling the powerful surge of the engine. He drives accompanied with the alarming knowledge that his patient's condition may be deteriorating by the minute. He presses the vehicle to the utmost: if the cops pick him up, he won't stop, he decides, he'll lead them into the hospital parking lot and settle with them later. Most likely they'll wave him on anyway, when they see the caduceus affixed to his licenseplate, he thinks hopefully. But maybe they're inured by now to seeing hospital-bound cars exceeding the speed limit in the vicinity of Memorial, but he hopes his theory won't be put to the test.

Within minutes Bairstow is on the last hill dipping into the hollow where the hospital is located. Fleetingly he glimpses his face in the rear-view mirror: his cocoa-brown hair, faintly tinged with premature gray, is standing in rumpled peaks, for he has a tendency to run his fingers through it when he's tense and worried, as he is now. He'd like to be certain at this minute that Emergency has acted efficiently to prepare this case, that they've responded with initiative and precision; in fact, that they've become clairvoyant in handling Helen Proctor-- but he senses that they may not have prepared so rapidly. He quickly combs back the tufts with the comb he keeps in a small tray under the dash, then looks fleetingly again at the face in the mirror: he's a handsome man, tan, fit, overworked--but he considers himself lucky in his profession, in his family, in his life. He's at the peak of his powers emotionally, professionally, and even financially and he knows it: this Lexus is a symbol of some of that, but Bairstow doesn't dwell on it--he's not a vain man, but he needs occasionally to reward himself for the 90 hours per week spent inside the gray hospital walls. He turns into the hospital's drive, lined with forsythia blooming, and slides into the hospital's reserved parking lot where his name is engraved on a neat metal plaque in one of the designated places.

The emergency room door flings open, and in a twinkling he's in his domain: beyond are the hushed corridors which can turn minute-by-minute into bedlam with the influx of torn accident victims, sobbing relatives, and screaming onlookers. Today everything is under control: Peggy Hagerty has been looking for him and hurriedly falls into step and begins to fill him in before he's hung up his coat. She is very quiet, her voice barely under control. "She's losing fast, Dr. Bairstow, blood pressure dropping like a stone. Oh, she knows what the trouble is, poor woman; she's smart as a cat, an uncanny lady." Peggy speaks still with a hint of an Irish accent, a light rhythmic lilt which has always made her speech sound musical to Bairstow's ears. Except for today, when the words are more forced and strained.

"Where is she, Peggy? She's conscious?" He can hear his own words, terse and taut.

Peggy nods and bites her lip, for she knows that the woman is barely conscious, that her life is slipping away, and that the woman knows it as well. Peggy leads Bairstow to Helen Proctor, back in the recesses of the emergency area, where the team has been working on her, one handling the cutdowns, another the oxygen, a third the blood. She's in a room of her own, now attended by another nurse while the operating room is prepared. Helen Proctor is lying on a gurney, ready to travel the route to the OR; already intravenous tubes snake in and out of her veins, and bottles dangle above her head, siphoning life-giving fluids into her body.

Bairstow is shocked by the woman's flaccid face, its waxen hue, and the glassy-eyed stare; he can remember the animated mien of the years when she was in active practice, the eager way she bustled about the wards administering to the patients. Now she is one herself, in need of the services of others. What she gave so freely to others must now return to her if she is to survive. Yet, as Bairstow contemplates her face, he doesn't make impassioned speeches to himself, "I will pull this woman through" or "We'll do it, one way or another," as he'd once done as an idealistic young surgeon. Now he knows better what he can do, that he can perform no miracles, but that his skill is far better than most. In the expertise scale of surgeons across the country, he rates himself at eight out of ten, and it is a solid judgment based on cool assessment. He has not the artistry of a Denton Cooley, Christian Barnard, or Michael DeBakey, but they are the virtuosos of his profession, and one cannot hope for that kind of superhuman skill without much training, a little luck, and sheer bravado. All those things Bairstow possesses in great degree, but he has never had the psychological compunction to face the world alone. He resists hype almost as much as he distrusts charlatans.

To his surprise, Helen Proctor raises her hand and smiles wanly, the corners of her eyes flicker...and Bairstow can see the spirit glimmering there as the woman looks straight at him. She is a fighter. To Bairstow that makes all the difference in the world.

"Take her up immediately," says Bairstow. "Ferraro's there?"

"Arrived five minutes ago, Dr. Bairstow. He said he'd be ready... about now." Peggy checks her watch. Ferraro, the anesthesiologist, is on call this weekend, too, and lives in the next block. Bairstow doesn't like him as well as Lehman, the other man, but it's mostly because Ferraro likes to brag about his golf scores even in the middle of surgery, and Bairstow worries that he isn't keeping his mind on his more urgent concerns. However, he's never had cause to doubt the man.

"Then let's roll." Bairstow goes on ahead while the aides transport the patient to the operating room. It's time for Bairstow to scrub. He enters the elevator to the surgical suite, which is hushed, muffled against contamination, pain and noise. The sounds of mortal combat, Bairstow's often thought, are quiet.

Jeff Potter has just arrived as well, and is ensconced in the doctors' surgical scrub room, brushing the thick suds up and down his hairy forearms. Jesus, we look like goddamed washerwomen, Bairstow thinks in a sudden revelation. Jeff is gowned in his greens, and now Bairstow removes his from its sterile package. In the operating room a nurse will cover him with another drape; it's part of OR procedure, the ritual since recent surgical time began, and has been second nature to Bairstow for so long now that he sometimes forgets that it's happening.

"They bumped the appendectomy?" Bairstow asks Potter.

Potter nods. He's blond, with fine features, a straight nose and ears set close to his head--a "pretty boy" in the envious description of Ferraro on occasion--but Potter takes it in good graces usually, telling Ferraro that "some of us have it and some of us don't." Yet it's entirely obvious that Potter doesn't relish being a "pretty boy" any more than Bairstow would, and that Potter would just as soon have made Ferraro's nose, already out of center, more lopsided on more than one occasion. "They called in the second team, Ben. It was Feldman's case. I guess he raised holy hell, but he didn't have much choice: that appendix wasn't going to kill the kid."

It's the first time that Bairstow knows he's bumped a kid--but he can't help that, either. Potter implies by his remark that he, too, is well aware that Helen Proctor might die of this complication to her heart valve, and that's the holy truth, also. Bairstow as yet has no idea what kind of mess he'll find inside the prone body of Helen Proctor.

He scrubs for three minutes instead of 10: he can see through the window into the operating room that Helen is being draped, and that Ferraro's begun the anesthesia. In this emergency, the niceties of surgical procedure will have to suffer. She is already limp, her body appropriated by others with her consent, entrusted in the hope that she may awaken cured. If the cure doesn't take, of course, she will never know the difference anyway...and perhaps she and Bairstow both think in the long scheme of things that's a blessing, although neither would admit to the thought.

Bairstow walks into the operating room followed by Potter. Both men hold their hands elevated to the air, and Charlotte Kirkham, head nurse on the case, slides on their gloves, the insides powdered to reduce the friction of their hands. Ferraro is preparing bags of blood for transfusion. They can hear Helen Proctor's slow breathing, amplified by the heart/lung machine. The room is freezing, to retard bacterial growth and slow the patient's living processes. Charlotte and Peggy Hagerty stand ready, deferential, patiently awaiting the beginning of the surgery. Before them lies the patient, her abdomen and thorax area still damp with the orange tincture painted over the operative surfaces. Bairstow stands on one side of the table and Potter on the other. The men are approximately the same height; otherwise the one assisting would accommodate himself by one device or another to the principal's stature; some short surgeons regularly stand on stools.

Bairstow lowers his head and begins the first incision. He feels himself more hurried, less careful than in the usual meticulously planned and plotted surgery--there's no time for it now. He learned textbook surgery in medical school and residency, his professors breathed rarefied air in the hallowed shrines of their closed circuit operating amphitheatres-- but many of those men, Bairstow feels, never lived in a real world where one deals with arteries in imminent danger of blowing. He bends over the incision, as do the nurses: they are clamping the blood vessels, not only to control blood loss, but to allow Bairstow to see what he's doing in the red welter of raw flesh.

Bairstow cuts again, this time deeper, then again. After mere minutes, the incision becomes a torrent of black blood as the last slice of flesh parts, and the torn aorta tumbles into the abdomen, freed of the pressure of the gut. "You've got enough blood ready for transfusion?" Bairstow demands of Ferraro, his voice betraying the urgency. He has a sudden realization of just how hairy this case is going to be, and feels immediately apprehensive, a rare transformation for him--and everyone in the room, sensing the momentary quaver, feels the urgency, too. He is instantly sorry that he betrayed even by inflection his doubt and gains prompt control, feeling calmed; he must keep those around him steady, too.

Ferraro nods. "They're ready, Ben."

Bairstow can feel the sympathy in the unaccustomed use by Ferraro of his first name; usually it's simply "Bairstow," or a statement with no name at all. Ferraro's nervous, too: that wound is a sobering sight, with its ropes of clot and brackish blood.

Bairstow is talking aloud, both to plan his course of attack and to alert Potter, who's holding a retractor and trying to make a judgment at the same time. Potter seems about to say something, but stops and looks at Bairstow, to see what he'll do next. There are obviously no set courses for this kind of thing.

"She's had a lot of previous surgery here," says Bairstow. "Look at these old adhesions, Potter. I'd say she's been opened three or four times before. I hope to hell the last guy left the renal artery well out of the way."

The two nurses glance at each other: the renal artery, they well know, is the vital main blood vessel to the kidneys.

Bairstow is moving more swiftly now. "We've got to get this area exposed," he tells Potter, his voice more urgent. "Move that retractor over here, can you?" He's concentrating on the field before him, on the mire of blood and tissue and the devastation caused by the strips of tissue from the former surgery. Potter has hastily set up one aspirator to pump out blood, but so far it isn't clearing the area: more blood is coming in than is being pumped out. The former nurse is deep in shock, close to death; Peggy Hagerty's voice quavers ever so little as she calls out the blood pressure readings: "60 over 40, Dr. Bairstow, pulse thready, pulse..." Bairstow knows one simple fact, and he's working against that knowledge: only so much blood can leave the system before pressure drops and the heart, with too little to pump, becomes disorganized and arrests. It's fundamental to all animals, and Bairstow knows that the time he has right now to save this woman is painfully, pitifully short.

Bairstow fleetingly wishes that he had a typical case before him now, when he could take time, when he could be painstaking, when the anesthesia could be meticulous and systematic and everyone in the room could perform his or her precise task precisely. Usually his surgery is not like this--this is far beyond what he's called on to accomplish in 98 percent of cases. His hands are submerged as he feels through the anatomy of the upper abdomen, groping for familiar organs as one in the dark searches for known structures and contours. He readjusts the automatic retractor which Peggy Hagerty has been struggling with and repositions it. "Watch it," he commands, and Peggy almost falls upon it as she fights her own panic. In the crisis Potter has grasped another retractor and holds back the gut for Bairstow and leans against it. The blown prosthesis is breaking up: it suddenly excretes a clot the size of a baby's fist, which floats up to full view. "Jesus Christ," says Potter, exhibiting emotion for the first time. "Will you look at *that*?" Blood floods into the widened incision.

"It's rupturing," says Bairstow, trying to remain cool, fighting for distance from panic himself. His hands are now sunk into blood to his wrists. Try as he can, he can't see what he's doing...and time is passing, precious, vital time. At least the transfusion is flowing. He has a moment of weakness, a minute of honesty so pure as to be almost ludicrous. "Unfortunately, damn it," he says, "my experience with this kind of complication is a little limited." It is the supreme candor, the moment of pure truth, the heart-wrenching reality of this instant to Ben Bairstow...and at that single instant, unlike earlier, his lapse causes not a flicker from Jefferson Potter nor the nurses. For Potter knows, as even the women suspect, that it is one surgeon in thousands who has the experience to deal with a complication like this, for patients who have aortic prostheses which rupture usually bleed to death in moments, and rarely get to the operating room table where help might await them. Only the fact that this woman is a nurse and savvy to her own life sounds has given her an edge on life; yet it is a doubtful edge at this moment. But Bairstow has, from long training, denied to his consciousness any real concession to imminent disaster: he works instead with possibilities, with probabilities, and with the skill one can muster, not with how he might fail. It is the only way he feels he can survive as a surgeon, there is no other. He must at all times live with hope.

He reaches vainly for surgical landmarks in the swampy murk before him; he can't even find the mouth of the flow so he can clamp it off. His fingers search desperately through the chaos of adhesions and clot, groping for something his mind can recognize, for a signpost, for anything familiar. Peggy pours saline solution into the wound to clear it, to sterilize it. The blood marbles, then reddens again. Potter is feeling about, too, searching for the elusive pulsing artery draining the patient's blood.

"Maybe..." says Potter after a minute, "just maybe..." He indicates a spot to Bairstow. Bairstow's hands rove toward the area.

"I don't know, Potter," says Bairstow. "I don't know." He looks away, trying to supersensitize his fingers, so they will *feel* with more acuity than they ever have before. The tension in the room is heavy, like a terrible ache. "I think I might have it, I just might..." He comes up with what he's grasped in his hands: it's the aorta's upper stump. He points to a large arterial clamp in front of Charlotte Kirkham. "I need a cooley, please, quickly." It feels as if no one has taken a breath for minutes. Denton Cooley's clamp, invented a half-continent away by the master surgeon, in Bairstow's hands just might save the day.

Peggy Hagerty gets a second aspirator operating at last, and after a minute blood begins to drain from the incision. The clamp comes into view as well as the tissues so long submerged, like a lost continent. The flow has come under control.

"If only I can get around the aorta, I can secure the clamp," Bairstow explains, mostly to Potter now. He was the man who'd found the stump, and his hand, still thrust into the woman's abdomen, keeps pressure on her organs, preventing the blood from leaving them. The patient's blood pressure begins to rise on the red digital meter beside her head: 57, 59, 65, 70, 80. The life force is returning within the nurse.

Bairstow begins to search for the remains of the old prosthesis, to remove it, pressing down with sugical pads at the same time to control the bleeding. "I can't tell if I'm feeling plastic or artery," he says. "Things are a real mess, a jumble." He thrusts with the clamp in his right hand, feeling it firmly in his fingers; in the left he holds scissors, opening the area tentatively as he goes, trying to find his way into new tissue.

"Maybe you're far enough," Potter suggests, peering into the area over his mask, at a different vantage point from Bairstow. "You might be in the real thing, above the old tissue. But I don't know..."

"I don't, either," answers Bairstow. But just then his fingers detect the ridge of the plastic, and he pulls it away and positions his clamp. "There, I've got it," he announces, his voice sounding almost triumphant. "That's it, I'm sure."

At the same time, everyone relaxes. Peggy looks at Charlotte and smiles. Potter eases the set of his shoulders.

"Syringe," says Bairstow, a little firmly now: he's noticed the relaxation and doesn't want too much of it. Peggy, guiltily, hands him the giant syringe with a bulb on the end. He draws up a cylinderful of blood, then returns it to Peggy, who squirts it into a bowl, placing into the bowl the new prosthesis which must be positioned to replace the defective plastic one.

"This is still spraying. Look at it, Potter," Bairstow says. "I've got it clamped, and we're still losing blood." He is now outraged at the recalcitrant organ, which is still failing to come under control despite all their best efforts. He studies the problem a moment longer, when another thought, equally alarming, occurs to him. "If this clamp is on the shreds of the old graft after all, and not back on the real aorta--and it blows along the old suture line--we're still in real trouble, Jeff. Damn, I can't seem to get any room to reclamp higher."

"Maybe I can help," says Potter. "I'll see if I can't clamp higher for you."

Both men probe into the wound deeper. At last the aspirator drains to the floor of the wound, so they can finally see the entire depth.

"It's okay," says Bairstow. "Thanks, Jeff." He slides in another arterial clamp and fastens it quickly just below the first. The spraying stops. Another release of tension. Now it's almost routine, the cleaning and tidying of the wound. Bairstow and Potter begin the process together, freeing strands of blood clot and pieces of debris from the blown prosthesis. "Neointima," says Bairstow, holding up some debris.

"Shit!" exclaims Potter. "Damned lot of crap."

Bairstow is used to Potter by now: he doesn't mind it when the younger man swears or indicates disgust. Bairstow wouldn't do it himself; he believes in professional decorum in the operating room and, in addition, respect for the woman on the table, as if she might hear. Disgust, Bairstow feels, is inappropriate for the human body. But in some ways he welcomes the release of tension in others. Bairstow trained in the days when the old Cushing school of surgery still exerted significant if waning influence, when the operating room was sancrosanct, and a little of that still controls him. Gross swearing bothers him anywhere, particularly in the OR, as if someone blasphemed in church.

Both men are silent for several minutes as they work to tidy the mess, like fastidious housewives. "There's the ring of the proximal aorta," says Bairstow: before him is a red cross-section of tube, craggy and rough-edged. "Like cement inside, and necrotic tissue outside. The poor woman almost bought it today for sure."

Potter leans forward to examine it more extensively, to observe his mentor's approach. Bairstow shows Potter how to do it, improvising his technique as he goes. He feels happy with Potter today: the man is young, but today he's been incalculably helpful. He's developing into a first-rate assistant, and will eventually become a first-rate surgeon as well. For now, in Bairstow's opinion, as a surgeon he's very good but not exceptional. "Please hand me a right angle, Peggy," Bairstow calls. He reaches into the aorta and fishes out more clot. Finding some, he probes farther. "That back wall is pretty eroded," he confides to Potter, "but we may have enough to work with." All the while he's talking, he's probing. Inches below the patient's pumping heart, Bairstow cleans the ring of the aorta, cutting it back to tissue stable enough to hold the new stitches which will tie in the new prosthesis: those stitches must hold in firm tissue or all is lost again.

Potter opens the incision into the belly farther under Bairstow's watchful eye. Give him a chance, Bairstow thinks to himself, he won't get a case like this again in a long while, and neither will I. There's a triumph about having saved the life of this woman, almost a confirmation of one's skills--that all those years of training worked. They've lost a few, too, Bairstow and Potter, but this time they succeeded. Salvation is sweet, for tomorrow may hold something else entirely. Together the two men inspect the lower section of the torn graft, their heads almost touching. Bairstow can smell Potter's sweat in this cool operating room over the usual scents of antiseptics and warm blood, forming a fulsome mix.

Bairstow clamps off the two iliac legs; the new graft, he decides in a moment of inspiration, would join not only the good aortic tissue at the top, but also the nylon cuffs at the bottom, thereby allowing for a smaller incision and a briefer operation. This patient, the old nurse Helen Proctor, has been through enough hell for one day.

Bairstow feels actual calm for the first time: sure, he's tried to give the aura of relaxed professionalism, but the mess inside this woman was almost too tough to sustain it. He signs almost audibly in relief. For a moment he wonders how Potter feels--but he's smelled Potter's sweat, and knows what it signifies. Bairstow moves slowly: he resets the retractors to open the wound farther; the two women keep the instruments coming, and they pull back the flesh when he asks. He chatters as he works, feeling buoyant that the worst is over, that he's in familiar territory.

Once Peggy Hagerty rubs against him; he wouldn't think anything of it except that she's done it several times before. It crosses his mind as he moves a retractor that it may not be a casual contact, that she's making advances to him--women have done it before. But he's always had a decent marriage. Mariam may not always have been a dynamo in bed, but she's a good mother and a devoted wife, and that's made up for a hell of a lot. Yes, there'd been a nurse once, very briefly, but he was not a man to throw himself around and it had not gone far. Miriam, to his knowledge, had never known.

"Peggy, two of us can't stand in the same spot at the same time," he says, gently but firmly when it happens again. "It's you or me. Do you want to take over this place?"

She looks at him, startled. "Sorry," she says, chagrined, moving away elaborately far. Bairstow thinks, she'll get over it, she's got better things to do in this operating room--then dismisses the whole thing from his mind.

"How're you doing over there, Ferraro?" Bairstow asks. "You haven't left for a coffee break, have you?" Ferraro hasn't spoken more than two sentences during the entire time of the surgery; he's sat behind his console monitoring the patient's vital signs and the ebb and flo of her life processes without blinking, it seems, as his anesthesia held her suspended from pain in her private limbo. Ferraro chuckles and shakes his head. "Still here, Ben."

"Well," says Bairstow, "I owe you one. Coffee afterward--this one has been pretty heavy."

"Big spender," says Ferraro, still smiling. Neither takes a drink on duty, though some men have been known to--but for them it'll be only coffee. But of the group surrounding his specialty, Bairstow sees Ferraro perhaps most often and knows the least about him: the man rarely talks. Bairstow's heard that he's saving to take a big trip sometime, to give up medical practice eventually, when he can afford it. He's been at Memorial for two years, plays good golf, and spends considerable time on a boat he owns. That's what he knows about Ferraro--almost as little as he knows about Potter.

"How're you doing, boss?" Charlotte Kirkham asks of Bairstow during a moment when he stops to change position and flex briefly.

"Just fine," answers Bairstow. "Thanks for asking. A great deal better than an hour ago."

Ferraro has come to life, and is reciting the vital signs more frequently. "The urine output has increased," he reports, uttering the words in a clear, singsong voice.

"The patient's or Bairstow's?" asks Potter.

Bairstow chuckles under his mask. It's time for a little lightness. On the whole, he thinks, it's been a successful case; they'd stood on the brink together, but they'd won.

CHAPTER TWO

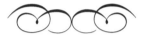

Bairstow had met Potter a brief three years earlier, when the younger man had applied for admission to the hospital staff and been accepted. After medical school he'd served his internship somewhere in the Midwest--it seemed to Bairstow that it had been Detroit. Now he's embarrassed to ask, because Potter has told him at least twice and he can't ask again. At any rate, he'd held his residency in New York, that much Bairstow can remember. Bairstow himself had gone to medical school, taken his internship, then followed it by his residency in Boston, so ordinarily he might not in the usual run of things have had much in common with a New Yorker, because medical affiliations seem to him something like clubs--but when Potter began to assist Bairstow, the two had hit upon an easy camaraderie. Occasionally Bairstow assists Potter in his surgery, although often other young men on the staff fill in with Bairstow. A kind of loyalty between the two men ensued, a give-and-take, supportive attitude toward the other, and a perception of the other's vulnerabilities. Bairstow will remember for a long while that Potter had found the loose end of the aorta in that bloody sump inside the patient's abdomen today. That kind of thing is worth a lot to Bairstow, and has already caused him to elevate Potter in the overall value he ascribes to their association.

After Helen Proctor is settled in the recovery room next door, Bairstow joins Potter in the dressing room adjacent to the operating suite. Bairstow is still wearing his green cap, having forgotten he has it on. Potter is shedding his scrub suit while Bairstow sits on a bench struggling with his shoes: they're a special kind, not only comfortable for long hours of standing, but constructed to eliminate static electricity, so no sparks will ignite volatile gases in the operating suite. Today they're slimed with Helen Proctor's blood.

"Gory spectacle," joshes Fred Abernathy, a staff gynecologist, observing Bairstow with mock distaste. Abernathy himself has just completed a hysterectomy and his operating suit is spotted with pale pink ooze, but it's virtually unblemished compared to Bairstow's. "Looks like we great healers are back again to blood-letting, Ben."

Bairstow nods; he can feel his fatigue setting in, although he's happy about his case. His patient will live to tell her grandchildren about this day, if she wishes to and they want to hear. At least he's restored her to a normal life expectancy, which is satisfaction enough.

"You, Potter?" Abernathy asks with a smile. "You've been assisting the great man?" Bairstow knows that it's all friendly banter and not calculated to annoy him, because he's been called the great man before, even within his earshot--but he still doesn't particularly like it. He prefers not to be singled out, though he knows that his surgery is beyond reproach and this case was calculated to test the will of even the steeliest of surgeons. He even recognizes that it's a kind of tribute, and as one of the more senior surgeons, he's bound to be treated deferentially by the younger crowd. Therefore, he accepts it in good grace.

"Aortic prosthesis blew," says Potter. "Godawful mess. Ask Bairstow, he stayed right with it. Couldn't even locate the damned stump for a while..."

"Really?" Abernathy's clearly astonished, his own routine surgery temporarily forgotten. "You found it? What did you do?"

"Put in a new one," says Bairstow. "Thought we'd lost the patient once, until Jeff put his finger in the rupture."

Potter turns to look at Bairstow: he's flattered by the senior surgeon's praise and had never expected it. During the time he's worked with Bairstow, he's found him professional and competent, but a little distant.

"If I hadn't found it, you would have," says Potter. "You know that's so, Bairstow."

"Maybe," answers Bairstow. "I certainly hope so. What are you up to, Fred?" Abernathy is shedding one surgical scrub suit and donning another.

"Another case, friend. You think I can just cut once and go home like you guys? I bet you've already read the funnies."

"Funnies?" Bairstow tries to act shocked. "You read the funnies, Fred? I would have guess the sports section, the editorials, maybe the stock market...but never the funnies!"

"Well...so I'm an addict. Wizard of Id, Doonesbury...that one with the dog. You name it, I read it. *Then* I read the sports page."

Bairstow refuses to acknowledge that he's already read the funnies and passed it along to his sons. "I'll bring you mine," says Bairstow. "I hate to see a good man deprived. It could lead to serious consequences."

"Glad you understand where I live," says Abernathy, who turns, waves, and walks through the door to an adjacent operating room.

For a moment Bairstow and Potter are silent, dressing. "You've got your new bike yet?" Bairstow finally asks Potter. It's the one thing about Potter that Bairstow knows: he's got an addiction to bicycle racing. For some time now he's been investigating new racing bikes, and he's been considering having one made.

Potter shakes his head. "It's the new European bikes that interest me," he says, becoming more animated. "They're more precise. Those moving parts are so finely honed that they never wear. I'm thinking of going into the big races."

"You mean, long distance riding?" Bairstow has never thought of Potter in that way--in fact, he's rarely thought of Potter outside the hospital at all. "You'd travel around the country?"

"Sure. On weekends. Like running, you know, you've got to go where they hold the big competitions."

Potter's energy puzzles yet fascinates Bairstow: had *he* been so energetic a mere ten years ago? Perhaps, but he's poured it all into his medical practice.

"What does your wife think?"

"June? She'll go along with anything I want."

"Really?" He makes a mental note to remember her name this time. June. "June's a racer, too?"

Potter laughs a little. "No, she stays home. She's a painter. She doesn't do much except paint."

Bairstow is undressing for the shower, his scrub suit already discarded. He tries to visualize what June Potter must be like to be married to a man who's gone on weekends, a woman who stays at home painting. He wonders what she paints.

"Sorry, you've never come to my house, have you?" continues Potter. "We'll ask you over sometime. Would you and Mrs. Bairstow come over if we asked you?" There's even hope in his voice.

"Miriam? Of course. It sounds like a nice idea...Jeff." Bairstow had been about to call him Potter, but you can't call a man by his last name if he's planning to invite you to dinner.

"Then I'll have June call. I'm off next weekend--and you are, too, aren't you? Or perhaps Kulick might cover, at least for a few hours, in case something comes up." Kulick is a general surgeon who sometimes spells one or the other for a few hours or even a day.

While Potter has been speaking, Bairstow is already in the shower, and waits until he's finished before answering, then pops his head through the curtain. "I'll be glad to check with Miriam, Jeff. She'll know what's on our schedule. I never have much of an idea myself, I'm afraid. Sometimes I think the world could stop out there and I'd never know it." It's a fact, and sometimes Bairstow has acknowledged to himself that what's happening out there seems insignificant as compared to the claustrophic life of this foolish institution.

Potter is preparing for his own shower: his towel is snugged about his waist. He has a lean look, Bairstow thinks, from all his riding. It makes Bairstow unconsciously flex his own biceps, as if to test their tensile strength; yes, they're still taut. Those days of football have endowed him with a well-muscled physique, and he still has it. I'm only 45, he thinks, I haven't exactly thrown in the towel. Maybe I'm even healthier than before, I eat well, and sleep...when I'm able. But I should get more exercise, I've got to do something about it. Now I'm even making lousy excuses for myself.

In street clothes: slacks, a shirt open at the neck, a navy sweater presented by the kids last Christmas, Bairstow stops to comb his hair, adjusting it so as to prevent a recalcitrant cowlick from thrusting an errant strand like a rooster tail off the back of his head. Then he detours briefly to see Helen Proctor, now in intensive care. She is the only patient there, guarded by two nurses. Helen is still unconscious, breathing easily, her color improved, the waxen, bloodless pallor having vanished when her pulsing aorta resumed its uninterrupted flow. Bairstow places his hand on her arm; the woman moves only sluggishly. Bairstow orders medication for her, then descends from the hospital wards to his car. Much has happened since he arrived at this place this morning, and his step feels a little lighter now than it would have if the case had gone less well.

He retraces his path home, this time in a less hurried fashion than when he arrived. The spring trees are budding, and forsythia bushes laden with blossoms are massed all along his route. This reminds Bairstow that he should call a gardener to feed his trees and shrubs or they'll end up as wan as last year, and lord knows he doesn't have time to tend them himself. Mirium either hadn't had the time to call someone to do the job last year, or there hadn't been anyone available to tackle the chore, but the yard *had* looked peaked--and he hadn't chosen a house with two acres of ground to let it turn drab. Maybe he should have taken a hand with the gardeners himself: it was true that sometimes people responded more readily to a man's voice than to a woman's, especially if it happened to be a doctor's. It puzzled him: do they respond to him because he's a man, or a doctor, or both? How do they respond to a woman doctor? He'll have to ask his female colleagues to check. But it seems highly unfair to Miriam. Yet time and time again he'd taken the phone and things clear away as if by magic. At least it's made his life, and Miriam's, easier. Of course, people are always telling him why they themselves haven't become doctors--oh, they'd considered it, almost gone for it, but at the last minute had opted for something else. Some had even told him that fact as if he, Bairstow, the dummy, the nitwit, had gone on to do this ridiculous thing of struggling through medical school, thereby blasting his mind and integrity for all time, when if he'd become a plumber his life would be easier and happier, too. So much for his foolishness. But then they go on at the same time to treat him with deference. It's very puzzling, but at least he is usually able to hire a gardener with aplomb--except for this year, it seems. Well, there is still time. Perhaps all the gardeners in his neighborhood who have almost gone to medical school are united in a front against people who have actually completed an education in such an indoor, unhealthy occupation (doctors breathe germs all the time, besides), and look down on the doctors as unwholesome types. Besides, it's not a good time for physicians--who'd want to be one on general principles?--because it seems everyone's suing them. Except that Bairstow had once thought he'd love to be a gardener; he loves puttering in the soil with plants and bushes, so perhaps if he communicated his fond wish to critics of doctors he'd be excused on general principles because they'd understand that his heart was in the right place.

His neighborhood is lovely, Bairstow thinks as he winds down the street. Herb Mathewson, who lives next door, has sunk enough manure into his rose bed and top dressing onto his lawn to turn a desert fertile; and glow it does, a veritable putting green, the grass gleaming with verdant ardor. Oh well, thinks Bairstow, not wanting to feel small-minded, even though he knows he's probably envious of Herb, at least my yard doesn't look prissy, as if all I do is tend petunias all day; Herb is retired, after all, and has more time to spend on his projects. Bairstow parks his car before his garage, attached to the long line of his house, not feeling like challenging the nonsequitors of his own argument. He feels a little tired and drained, but he's home.

"It's you, Ben?" Miriam asks, calling from the kitchen where she's preparing dinner. He can see her figure through the window, vaguely concealed by the reflection of the glass. Her dark hair is brushed delicately with gray, and she has a good figure despite three kids. Bairstow knows he's still attracted to her sexually: sometimes the mere sound of her voice on the telephone gives him an erection, especially when he's been away at a medical meeting and he yearns for her. Their 19-year marriage has been a good one. Her father had been an attorney in Concord, the state capital of New Hampshire, made a little money, and held an exalted opinion of himself, at least in Bairstow's estimation. When he died three years ago, the family felt his loss and wept for him, but at least they no longer had to put up with his querulous lectures at family gatherings about money or politics. When he'd thought about it afterward, Bairstow discovered that he really had little affection for his wife's father--but Miriam's mother lives on--more happily, it seems to all who know her--playing bridge with her friends without the constant surveillance of her overbearing spouse. Miriam, Bairstow also noted, now has a tendency to visit with her mother more, either in the old family home in the mountains--or the older woman drives down to see them here in Tennafield, Massachusetts.

Bairstow opens the door of his house and lays his sweater across the chair in the den: Sunday is far from over, and he may have to dash for the hospital again in the course of the day. At night when he's on call he arranges his essential belongings, even socks, on the chair in the living room, where it's warmer to dress, for that moment when the call comes and he has to awaken, sleepy-eyed, and depart like a cannon shot for the emergency room. At least the ride to the hospital wakes him up, allowing him to collect his wits. He knows that when he's inside the pneumatic doors of his place of work, he's supposed to appear in charge of himself, the compleat physician, and he doesn't want to disillusion anyone by appearing in mismatched clothing.

"You're back," says Miriam: it's an obvious fact, but Bairstow knows it's meant in a larger connotation, that he's back mentally, too, even emotionally, in the sense that he's home. "How'd it go?"

He shrugs, not really wanting to go into it. "Got her stitched together, Mimi, guess that's the important thing." Years ago, when they'd seemed too formal on their first dates, Bairstow had jokingly called her Mimi, and as their relationship ripened, the name had stuck. Miriam had liked the lightness of it, after all those dour years of her upbringing. Her father had hated it: what was wrong with Miriam, her given name, he'd demand of Miriam's mother, and the woman had reported it to Miriam with a smile, as though she were secretly pleased they'd done something on their own without consulting the old curmudgeon.

Bairstow kisses Miriam on the forehead, then helps himself to a small, delicate tart, dusted with confectioners' sugar, which still lingers on the baking sheet before him. He takes a bite, shakes his head, then reaches for another; each is a mouthful of confection, covered with a gossamer web of sugar. "How do you expect me to stay trim," he says, thumping his midriff, "if you bake things like that for dinner?"

"Actually," says Miriam with a grin, "they're for the bridge club, but what they don't know won't hurt a bit."

Bairstow smiles back, waves his hand, then strolls out through the open door toward the yard where the lawn chair he'd set up before the sprint to the hospital still awaits him. The Sunday papers (largely untouched except for the funnies which are missing and undoubtedly demolished by now by the twins) are still furled in two folded masses of newsprint. What a stand of trees, Bairstow thinks, must go into these two Sunday metropolitan editions we read each week! Why, it must take an entire forest for this single day's outout. The same thought has been occurring to him for some time now, since he read an article about the deforestation occurring in this hemisphere during the past few years...and for a while he even felt guilty about it. But finally he let it go, because if one sat down to worry about all the things one can't control, how would one carry on with the normal cares of a life, anyway? Why, he'd argued logically, it would cease to be manageable at all, those things to which one owed allegiance, and one might even falter under the burden and strain of struggling with them and end up in the forgotten back ward of some dismal institution somewhere?

He eases back into the chair and begins to read the financial page: some of his stocks, particularly the foreign ones, are actually rising after a bad period. He's never considered his assets as anything especially associated with him, feeling they have more to do with his accountant, who phones now and then to swap stories and recommend he hold onto this one and sell another. His accountant, a fussy little man who habitually wears a bow tie--perhaps he sleeps in it, too--obviously loves the give and take of this kind of thing and for this Bairstow is happy because he doesn't, and is grateful for the occasional exchange. Bairstow has stocks in a mutual fund and in a few bonds and in silver and gold as well as a high-risk account which his accountant has warned him about and even indicated his stern disapproval, but he has given up protesting because Bairstow is Bairstow and savors a little risk. Bairstow is not particularly well-heeled, as some doctors with more investment know-how are, partly because of his tendency to risk money but also because he decided rather late to set up some kind of program. He feels that the Lexus is really the only affluent symbol he cares to maintain. He knows men who have dropped dead at his age, so he carries good life insurance for Miriam and the kids. Actually he's a man who hates to think about money because it bores him stiff, and he can't really imagine what fun a stockbroker gets out of life. But he has a tender spot for other kinds of toiling people: steelworkers who work arduously in hot plants, coal miners who labor so far underground, mailmen (although he can't quite think why, perhaps it's because they get attacked by dogs, and he's never particularly liked dogs), steeplejacks, and repair people because they repair plumbing as he does in his own business. He admires, besides gardeners, truck drivers, salesmen, and hockey players. He's inclined to revere motion, stamina, and dedication, and he feels that all of the former qualify in some category or other. Of course, some of those professional skills apply to his own field as well, perhaps even that of salesman, for Bairstow must frequently sell some pretty tough diagnoses and treatments to recalcitrant patients, and if he hadn't entered this business of medicine, could conceivably have been a success selling advertising campaigns to skeptical soap manufacturers. He cocks his head at the notion. Well, maybe not.

After ten minutes, he's restless, and moves across the lawn to the greenhouse. He had it built when the house was completed six years ago as a kind of afterthought, thinking that he might have spare time to tend a garden year-round. And for a while that first year before patients got to know him, he *had* found time to grow, fertilize, and nurture a few plants--before his surgery took off on its frantic pace. Now only Miriam keeps a few motley houseplants on its shelves which she's coaxing back to life from winter doldrums. Last fall the twins had incubated a litter of kittens in its sunny warmth when Victoria had decided to spawn on the rug behind the couch, but was persuaded that a nest in the greenhouse would do as well. The kittens have long since been doled out to willing neighbors and the cat spayed (for a while Bairstow had been tempted to perform the job himself when he heard the veterinary fees, but had been dissuaded by Miriam and the boys in a loud, vociferous howl of disapproval). Perhaps that was for the best, he'd reflected afterward, cat anatomy not being his forte now as it had been so long ago when he'd become involved so intimately wiith comparative anatomy in college.

I'll have to get this greenhouse going again, Bairstow thinks as he walks through empty potting tables for which he'd held such high hopes. Disused wooden flats, some of them green with mold, are stacked in a corner, and potting soil in bags stands on the floor, Miriam still using the loam for her garden plants. A trowel layered with damp peatmoss rests on a table. Hanging begonias being lured back to health and to blossom hang in one corner, suspended by hooks from the metal frame. If only there were time, Bairstow thinks, maybe he could begin here again--but that's been the problem all along, time, and he doesn't want to challenge its supremacy until he gets older and things slacken off a bit, if that ever occurs.

Restless still, Bairstow returns to the house, to stand in the door and talk to Miriam. Stirring spoon in hand, she turns to face him. "Well?" she asks with a smile. "What now?"

"Potter's invited us to dinner," he says, leaning against the jamb. "Next Saturday. His wife will call. What are we doing?"

Miriam consults her calendar behind the pantry door. Bairstow notices that she has a spot of confectioner's sugar on her cheek, and steps inside to wipe it off with a finger. "Nothing," she says. "You mean Potter? You're sure he means dinner?"

"I know. He's never asked us before. But I'd like to go. It suddenly dawned on me how little I know about the man, and I scrub with him almost every day."

Miriam nods, even if she doesn't understand this man she's been married to for lo, these many years, who's taken to sudden whims like going out on Saturday, then won't budge from his chair for weeks on end for any social occasion at all unless she coaxes.

"Then let's go," she says. "You've met Dr. Potter's wife?" She always refers deferentially to her husband's colleagues, not wishing to use her favored position as a doctor's wife to act with familiarity.

"Never. Her name is June, that's all I know. They don't have any children. By the way, where are Norman and Pete?"

"Brody's. They've gone to the cottage, to open the place up for the summer. They asked our kids along."

"You mean, to clean it up?" Obviously the Brodys never inspected their kids' rooms.

Miriam smiles, the friendly lines about her eyes deepening. "Kids don't willingly clean their *own* rooms, Ben, they only do it at our insistence. Don't you know that by now?"

Bairstow shakes his head wonderingly. "Then maybe we should hire them out, Mimi. We might even make quite a profit with all that new-found cleaning energy. My mother used to make me clean *my* room." Then he wishes he hadn't said that, because he hadn't meant it as a criticism of Miriam. Yet sometimes Bairstow has thought she *wasn't* firm enough, that occasionally the kids got away with murder. And now there's that problem with Amanda, caught shoplifting a bra and panties at the department store last month, when she has a drawerful at home. So his own daughter had to come home to face them for her crime, as well as confront the judge, who told her in no uncertain terms what she must do to redeem herself in the eye of the law: pay the fine of $1000 or go to jail on this first offense. Maybe if they'd both been firmer as parents, he thinks, or more perceptive, she'd have turned out better. Now, perhaps prep school can straighten her out, who knows? Which came first, he's wondered, the innate tendency of a person to steal or the parents' mistake of omission in raising one's child so that she stole? Both resulted in the same transgression, so how was one to know? Bairstow doubts he'll even discover the answer, but the question, the mere act of asking it, frustrates and leaves him drained because there's nowhere to go with it. It's a total non-sequitur. Except that Amanda will have to earn the fine herself--no way is he going to pay it—and he's instructed Miriam to take more control of Amanda's comings and goings

But Miriam, annoyed and shocked as she is with Amanda, merely seems introspective today. "I agree entirely," she says, her thought processes paralleling Bairstow's as they often do, "that I should have landed a little more solidly on Amanda. "But *my* mother never intimidated me, either, Ben, you know that. She was too busy fending off my father."

It's true, Bairstow thinks--Miriam's description is an exact one of her own home life. Somehow, somewhere, Amanda derived her own idea of how the world functions--Miriam doesn't have to feel responsible. Miriam is a good woman, she's generous to her friends and to her family as well. They tried to treat Amanda fairly, and she stole. There's no way for him to assess that, and Miriam can't, either.

"Forget it," says Bairstow apologetically, waving his hand as if to recapture his flown words. "That's not what I meant, anyway. By the way, when *does* Amanda get home from prep school?" Miriam is the one who takes care of these details: she knows where the children are, when they will return, who they see, what they do, within reason, excerpt on Amanda's recent shopping trip. Sometimes, Bairstow thinks, he must seem a mere ship passing in the night, but he can't help it.

"Next week, first time since the hearing. Apparently she's been waiting table weekends at the Ramada to satisfy the fine, at least that's what her roommate said. It keeps her busy and out of trouble. I hope."

The understatement of the year: can the young daughter of a halfway prominent family who has copped a plea for shoplifting ever be gainfully employed again? Maybe so, but it sounds like a damned soap opera. Perhaps the counseling has helped: Amanda, twice a week, sees a counselor. Bairstow pays the bills. There's a terrific arrangement, Bairstow thinks with annoyance, even though he tries to keep his feelings to himself. At least she goes, which is the best thing of all.

Bairstow turns and walks back out into the sun to read the rest of the paper. It's a rare moment: he has the entire yard to himself, he'll take advantage of the peace and quiet, at least until he gets called out again. He may have five minutes, 50 minutes, five hours. His life is precariously uncertain, his time to himself prescribed: within a half-hour he could be back inside the operating room, stitching up a perforated bowel or a bleeding ulcer or heart valve, God forbid--one today was enough to last him a while. Sometimes he thinks he sits on a very precarious balance, at an apex from which he could fall at any time, but he likes the uncertainty of this profession, he chose it, and somehow the imponderables of his world give him confidence to surge forward, they run with his own inner clock or tide or whatever it is that governs him. It is fitting that his business should dovetail with his own ebb and flo in this mysterious way which he can't begin to comprehend to his own satisfaction and could never describe to anyone, not even Miriam.

He picks up the newspaper again, this time the book review, and begins to read. In 10 minutes he's asleep, the sun aslant his face. Miriam looks out at him through the kitchen window; he looks content, she thinks, when he's relaxed this way, more like the man she married. Lately he seems tense and restless, but he's always pushed himself and relished the demanding world he lives in, and she knows she has no real control over him nor would she want any. She knows that they've been after him to take over as chief of the surgical staff, which would make more claims on him by far, involving as it does additional paperwork along with the prestige. Miriam is aware that her husband is a good surgeon, even an excellent one...and also a man unto himself who will not communicate where he wants to go until he's taken the first step. He's always been that way. Her father had been a private man, too, but almost a stealthy one, a perverse character who liked to bait others with his obstinacy. Ben is not like him--he's humane and kindly, sparing of others, but determined and essentially a loner.

Yet, she thinks as she looks at him through the glass, he seems to be going through something, perhaps a time in his life which stands out unlike any other, something which is arresting in his own destiny. Maybe he doesn't know it himself, but she does. He seemed fitful, prowling around in the greenhouse that way. This is the first time he's been still since he arrived home. Soon the damned phone will ring again, and he'll be gone. Things seem to be crowding around both of them lately--with Amanda coming home. Well, time will tell; somehow resolution of sorts will come about for all this, she thinks philosophically. She'll have to hope for the best.

She carefully puts her tarts into a tin box and snaps on the lid.

CHAPTER THREE

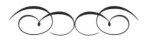

As Bairstow sits in the chair on his lawn, he dreams: he can see himself clearly as a kid. He was a sturdy boy with bandaids on his knees because his mother thought the bandaids were more sightly than the scrapes and subsequent scabs. Bairstow himself preferred the scabs; they seemed somehow more ennobling than the pristine white plastic strips, and he'd remove the bandaids as soon as he escaped from home. He didn't actually defy his mother, but she wasn't a disciplinarian, and he could usually get away with anything he wanted. He can see himself now as he dreams, contemplating a climb to the top of a tree between his house and school--it was a tree higher than any of the other boys were willing to climb, and Bairstow had acquired a certain fame for his daring. Yet when he'd looked up that day with all the other boys watching, he can still recall his terror; he was only ten. Yet he remembers it clearly, dreams it as if it were this morning, or yesterday, or last week. He'd contemplated that tree beforehand, planning how he'd conquer it; later, determined, he'd taken a deep breath, then shinnied his way to the very top, his body a tense spring. But, to his surprise, he'd found himself relaxing as he climbed higher and higher. He can remember glimpsing the boys down below watching, having fallen silent as they contemplated the form of their comrade inching skyward. When Bairstow had finally reached the topmost crown of branches, he hadn't bothered to look down again or even wave; instead he'd gazed about the incredible landscape visible from that height--at the broad band of the Connecticut River beyond the western hills, at the roofs of the houses below, and the precise geometric green of the park a half-mile away. He decided that very day, at that very moment in fact, far above the earth as he contemplated his singular feat, that he wanted to become a doctor, that he dared to aspire to it. He knew it now. He'd actually been thinking of it for a while since the day the family doctor, Dr. Enslip, had been consulted to cure his strep throat. Bairstow had felt an instant allegiance to the office of Dr. Enslip that day a year ago, not only because the doctor's ministrations had enabled him to return to climbing trees, but because he loved the smell and colors of the tinctures, the lure of the strange vials and various instruments, and the personality of Dr. Enslip as well.

Bairstow can picture him now: a short, craggy, bearded man with faded blue eyes--uncommunicative but scrupulousy honest-- who refused to dispense even placebos if they did the patient no good. He had absolutely no faith in psychological medicine. He also had no faith in most of his colleagues, and sometimes said as much, which frequently ostracized him from county medical meetings. But that day something had occurred in Dr. Enslip's office which Bairstow could only acknowledge far up in the solitude of that tree: he would follow Dr. Enslip's profession and do what he did. He saw that decision from 50 feet in the air with utmost clarity and unshakable commitment.

Bairstow awakens, knowing instantly what his dream had been about because for some reason he'd been dreaming it a lot lately. He reflects on the life he's led but finds himself uneasy: on the whole he doesn't much like thinking of the past. But if he reexamines it, he reasons, perhaps his dream will go away, like temporary indigestion. If, like a dyspeptic, he discovers it's merely fresh strawberries ruining his sleep, he'll know to eliminate the strawberries. Maybe he's working too hard, but he's always worked hard. His father had been a workaholic, foreman of the tooling plant where he was employed. He reported to the factory early, late, and on weekends. Just like me, thinks Bairstow, we're cut from the same damned cloth. His father's absence from the home left him, the oldest son, not even a teenager yet, with responsibilities far beyond his years. It was the making of me, Bairstow has thought on more than one occasion: he'd take the family money and go shopping with it on Saturdays for all the staples they would need during the coming week. For years his mother had been ill, steadily wasting away, and now he knows that she probably had some sort of sclerosis, probably amyotrophic lateral. Although young, he looked older because he was taller and stronger than most children in the neighborhood. His position of eldest of four offspring gave him, besides stature, a certain aura of maturity, whether he had it or not. If he experienced little formal family structure, he also had freedom: other kids had to wear their shoes and wipe their noses and account for their time away from home, but not Bairstow. The only penalty was those damned bandaids.

As Bairstow sits in the chair on his lawn, he can see another face besides that of Dr. Enslip's and his parents: Father Grogan's. Bairstow was educated in parochial school and was the top student in his class in high school. It came easily, he didn't even have to work hard. Father Grogan, he thinks now, leaning his head back to conjure up the priest, was an ardent, dedicated Catholic who desperately wanted him to join the order. Once, Father Grogan had informed him in the off-hand manner he had, that the four top students of the last three classes had already declared their allegiances to the priesthood, and Bairstow understood that day in the corridor of the parochial school what Father Grogan had designated him to do. But Bairstow already knew he wanted medicine, not Catholicism: he'd emerged from that tree a changed boy. But he didn't want to inform Father Grogan just yet.

"But...I'm not religious enough," Bairstow had stammered to Father Grogan that day. "Maybe, if only I felt more...holy, or worthy or something, but I don't."

Father Grogan had placed his hand on Bairstow's shoulder. "You will change, Benjamin. When the spirit of our Lord enters your soul..."

Bairstow could feel himself squirming, because it hadn't entered yet and he was virtually certain it never would if it hadn't done so by now. He shook his head discreetly, having no wish to antagonize the priest. "Thank you, Father, I'll think about it."

"I hope you do, young man. You know the aspirations of the human soul: the Good, the Beautiful, the True. Naturally those should be your aspirations as well, and your life directed along more exalted lines..."

The Good, Beautiful and True gave Bairstow a headache because they were so formidable to think about, almost terrifying. He couldn't comprehend them, deal with them, or contemplate what they were all about because he couldn't even picture them in his mind except as foggy, dark, frightening shapes. Besides, what was so wrong with wanting to be a doctor?

He rarely dated as he grew older, because somehow he had the idea that it was frowned on, too, though in his junior year he had a crush on a redheaded girl in his English class named Sally Stearn. He walked home with her for a while though she lived a distance from his neighborhood, until it took too much time from his responsibilities at home: his mother was growing weaker by the day, and the demands on Bairstow had increased. So he met with Sally at school, sitting on the stone steps behind the classroom building, until he realized that Father Grogan and the others had noticed. Bairstow was called again to the priest's office.

"Have you reconsidered yet, Benjamin?" Father Grogan asked.

"Reconsidered?" Yet Bairstow wasn't entirely ignorant of the Father's purpose.

"You haven't indicated yet whether you wish to become one of us. I thought we would have heard by now."

Bairstow didn't wish to hurt Father Grogan's aspirations for him, but he didn't want to be a priest, either. "I'm sorry, Father, but I have other plans."

"Other plans? What other plans? What could those plans possibly be that they are more important than the priesthood?"

"I want to be a doctor, Father. I told you. I've been thinking about it for a while now."

"A doctor? You think being a doctor is more worthy than...?"

"I don't know about *worthy*, Father. I only know that's what I want to do." All along Bairstow had thought that Father Grogan would be pleased, because no one had ever graduated from this school to become a doctor.

"Well, you still have time to change your mind," said Father Grogan, his dark eyebrows almost touching in his displeasure. "We hate to lose a boy. We'll speak of it again."

Bairstow had joined the yearbook because Sally Stearn worked on the staff. By the end of the year he was elected feature editor. "You'll be made editor-in-chief, Ben, I'm sure of it," said Sally enthusiastically, with great conviction. "You really are good, you know."

The flattery from Sally rather than the thought of making editor inspired Bairstow to redouble his efforts to succeed on the staff. He spent extra time on his copy (especially when Sally was also in the newsroom), and took pains that it be clean and clear. The time in spring was approaching for the staff to make plans for the following year: it was to be Bairstow's senior year and he could hardly wait. "You'll make it for sure," said Sally. "No one is as good or as conscientious as you are."

Father Grogan summoned him after class one day to his office on the top floor of the main classroom building. It was a resplendent office, with a Persian carpet on the floor, a large, carved mahogany desk behind which Father Grogan stood as Bairstow entered the room, leaded windows, high ceilings, and ecclesiastic oil paintings across the walls. It was in sharp contrast to the school, which was spartan and drab.

"How's it going, Benjamin?" the priest asked him. "We have given you time to reconsider, I think. I've told you, our first students have always come into the order. Your senior year is coming right up."

"Yes, Father."

"You will follow us and join, then, to become one of us?"

"N...no, I've already told you what I want to do. I *really* want to become a doctor."

Grogan had rubbed at his cheek impatiently. "I'd hoped you might have given that up by now. I had more faith in you than that."

"I'll never give it up, sir."

"In spite of what I've just been saying to you, of my prayers for you?"

Bairstow had no idea that he'd been in Father Grogan's prayers. "Yes, Father, I've made up my mind."

Father Grogan had been standing, but now he sat down behind his desk, leaving Bairstow to stand alone. He fiddled with a pen on his desk; on the top, Bairstow saw, was a tiny replica of the crucifix. "I understand, Benjamin, that you're running for the position of editor-in-chief of the yearbook."

"Yes, sir, I..."

"Don't you think that office should go to one with deeper religious conviction than yours? To a person who professes a truly spiritual nature, who takes our church and our order more seriously?"

Even now Bairstow can feel the humiliation of the priest's words: they sting and rankle whenever he remembers them. He'd never heard of a person who insulted a priest or showed discourtesy to a nun for that matter, and he never could act disrespectfully to this man of the cloth. But it all seemed so terribly, terribly unfair somehow. He tried to control himself as best he could. "I'm sorry, Father, if you don't think I take the church seriously. I do, I really do, honest. But that doesn't have anything to do with my being a doctor. Why, lots of doctors respect their churches..." He was almost in tears.

"You don't need to lecture me, Benjamin. But I wouldn't apply for the position on the yearbook if I were you. This parish makes its *own* decisions about officers among the student body, and all candidates must be approved by a...select group. I head the group. Of course, if you should change your mind about joining the order..."

Bairstow, stung, had turned and walked from Father Grogan's office. He didn't run for the office of editor-in-chief, and a man farther down on the editorial staff was selected.

Sally Stearn was incredulous. "I don't believe that happened to you," she muttered over and over when Bairstow told her. "Why, that was cruel, Ben. I never though Father Grogan could ever be so mean."

"Neither did I, Sally. But when I get out of here, I'll never have anything to do with this church ever again, I swear it."

"Please don't say that, Ben. Father Grogan isn't everyone."

Bairstow had turned his back to the school building. "I can't help it, I've had enough of this place to last me forever. Maybe I'll even become a heathen."

He'd meant it as a joke, but he could see that it had wounded Sally. He quit the yearbook staff and stayed away from all extracurricular activities the school offered. He saw Sally only rarely after that, not only because of the way he felt about the school, but because he also knew that Sally was a loyal Catholic who basically disapproved of his action. Besides, his mother had become increasingly unwell and needed his help.

During the summer before senior year, his mother died: she simply wasted away. Bairstow's younger sisters cared for her while he worked at the local gas station pumping gas to help his father pay for medicines and visits to Dr. Enslip. When he had an extra few minutes, he helped the mechanic repair cars, because if he were to carry out the dream formulating in his head, he'd need money, and it was more profitable to repair cars than to fill their tanks.

His dream was to go to Harvard after he graduated, a year away--and while he knew it was crazy for him to think about it, he was determined to try. No one else in the family had completed high school, much less college, much less Harvard. He didn't tell anyone because it sounded so impossible. But Dr. Enslip *had* gone to Harvard, and on a visit to his mother, the doctor told Bairstow that if he worked hard enough, just maybe he'd get there. When Bairstow confided that he was at the top of his class scholastically, Dr. Enslip said he'd write a letter of recommendation for him, that he didn't see why a bright boy like Ben wouldn't make it, but not to count on anything, just the same.

When Bairstow's mother died, it was a devastating time for him because he'd loved her dearly, but he continued pumping gas and learning from the mechanic. At the end of the summer he'd saved some money but not enough for even one year of college, so he wangled a job to continue working after school for his entire senior year. He liked the work and it helped relieve the painful memories of his mother's death and the humiliation he'd suffered at the hands of Father Grogan.

But one obstacle remained, and Bairstow judged it to be a minor one: late in the fall he had to ask the school to forward his records to Harvard if he were to apply for admission there. Bairstow thought it was routine, that he merely had to request the transcripts from the office. Once more Bairstow was summoned to Father Grogan's office. This time the priest again remained seated.

"I understand you want your records forwarded, Benjamin. Where did you want them sent?"

"Harvard, Father. That's where I'm applying."

"Not a Catholic school, is it? Why not Boston College?"

"Because I don't want to go to Boston College. I want to go to Harvard." This time Bairstow was determined not to let the priest put him down.

"Then we won't forward your records. We are not in the business of sending records to schools we don't sponsor. And we won't recommend you, either,"

Bairstow had to fight for control. "Then I'll do it on my own. I'll go to Harvard, you wait and see. I don't want one of your schools, ever. Not ever!" He'd been about to add that he'd never again set foot inside a Catholic church, but he did have a few more months of education to endure and he didn't want his grades tampered with. Besides, he realized that this miserable priest didn't represent the entire hierarchy of his faith.

Father Grogan merely looked at him and didn't even bother to answer. He waved his hand for Bairstow to leave, and somehow that wave, Bairstow thought afterward, was meant as a dismissal from an entire way of life, from the world he'd grown up in. It signified that from that time on, Bairstow was on his own. True to his word, Father Grogan refused to allow the transcript to be sent out. Bairstow decided to journey to Harvard on his own, to talk to the admissions people. It was what Dr. Enslip suggested that Bairstow do, and when Bairstow left for Cambridge, he carried a letter of recommendation from the doctor in his pocket.

Bairstow had been to Boston with his father once before on a mill convention, but not to Harvard. He was impressed by the graceful stone buildings along the Charles River, but not overawed. This is where he intended to go, after all, and he saw it as a flesh-and-blood place where he had to gain admittance. He wasn't entirely convinced that Harvard wanted in its ranks a poor boy from the hinterlands whose school wouldn't even corroborate his academic record. But, luckily, Bairstow's mother had saved his old report cards, virtually all he'd received from grade school on, and Bairstow carried those along with what records he could recover of his sports and extracurricular activities, carefully preserved in a plastic folder he'd purchased at the local dry goods store.

When the secretary at the admissions office looked him over, a little startled, Bairstow glanced down at his clothes and saw the old knickers, neatly darned (his church pants, if he should ever go again) and new socks in old but polished shoes. He was wearing his best sweater, but it, too, was faded. Perhaps, he thought, he should have gone out to buy a new suit, but then he wouldn't have had enough money to make the trip to Cambridge. Besides, he didn't know what academics had to do with the way you looked: sartorial splendor wasn't a goal in his young life. But he began to feel that he might have made a big mistake when he saw the director of admissions looking at him a little oddly, too.

"You want to come to Harvard?" the director asked. "Why is that your ambition, young man?"

"Because it's the best school there is. And I want to go to medical school afterward, I've already decided. I have a letter, you see here"... Bairstow opened his plastic case..."from a friend who's a doctor. He recommended me." Bairstow placed on the director's desk the stack of report cards, tied with blue ribbon, and the letter.

If the director was astonished, Bairstow thinks now, he tried to conceal it. "I see. We have your letter in our files requesting this interview, but nothing from your school. You didn't ask them to send on your records?"

This, of course, was the obstacle, and Bairstow had to face it as best he could. "They won't send my transcripts. Father Grogan says...." For a minute Bairstow couldn't continue, because it sounded so absurd that his school wouldn't help him in any way, in fact was diametrically opposed to his admission.

"Yes?"

"My school wants me to go to a Catholic college. I attend a parochial school. They refused to send my records to Harvard."

The director looked even more astonished: he'd encountered this kind of thing before, but it still amazed him. "That's why you brought along your report cards? It was a wise thing to do. The only thing, under the circumstances."

The director questioned him for a few more minutes, then sent him to a dean, one of the other members of the admissions committee. Bairstow repeated his answers to the director's questions, received a pat on the back, then went back out into the cold, for it was fall and a cold wind was blowing from the water. He watched the boats on the Charles River, then boarded a trolley and began the journey home. In time he was accepted at Harvard, and never had to appear before Father Grogan again except once, when he graduated. Bairstow shook his cool hand; Father Grogan offered no word of congratulation despite the fact that Bairstow was second in his class. A "good Catholic boy," as Father Grogan characterized him, had copped first place. Bairstow was only glad that he hadn't been demoted farther down the list for his heresy. But he didn't really care, because he carried his letter of acceptance from Harvard in his pocket on the day he graduated.

A few years later when he was visiting the home of a friend who'd gone to the same parochial school, Bairstow noticed on the coffee table an issue of the yearbook that he himself had once worked on as a staff member. He picked it up, gingerly, as if there still might be pain in it. As luck would have it, it was the graduation issue, and prominently displayed on the front page was the picture of a boy who'd just been accepted at Harvard. Bairstow held the issue closer, reading the print. "The first in the history of the school to get into Harvard," he read. "The school is proud of his excellence."

Bairstow had let the paper drop to the floor, as if it were contaminated. Maybe the school has changed, he thought, but that man surely wasn't the first to get into Harvard. He wondered for the first time what had happened to Father Grogan, but didn't really care. Bairstow hadn't stepped into a church in years; by then he'd finished Harvard College and Harvard Medical School and had decided to become a surgeon. He was also dating a woman named Miriam Lockland, who was also Catholic and they were talking of being married in the Catholic church, so Bairstow thought that perhaps things *do* come full cycle. But at least he'd never set foot again in the old school.

Bairstow and Miriam *did* marry in the Catholic Church, which caused Bairstow conflict--but he realized that his skin was tougher than it used to be. Now he attends occasional church services only for Miriam's sake and never goes to confession. Miriam complains occasionally that she "can't get through to him" about becoming a practicing Catholic once again, but she doesn't badger him because she knows that when he's made up his mind she can't change it.

Once his college roommate during their second year at medical school suggested he submit to psychoanalysis--the roommate himself, having decided to specialize in psychiatry, was departing every morning for a visit with his shrink before setting off for classes. He felt that everyone should be analyzed at one time or another. Bairstow staunchly refused. Now and then Bairstow still sees his roommate, who has a successful psychiatric practice.. But during that medical school year the man had become so moody that he was almost impossible to live with, and Bairstow thought: if that's what happens when you start to look inside yourself, I want no part of it. Maybe it's best to keep a distance from your inner thoughts and doubts. At least that's what he'd rationalized: you're bound to get into trouble, he'd thought, when you start to question everything you do.

CHAPTER FOUR

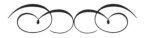

The Potters live in a modern house on an acre of land in the woods. That surprises both Miriam and Bairstow. Somehow Bairstow had thought of Jeff in a smaller house in a nice suburban development, but he can't say why. Jeff opens the door for Miriam and Bairstow, but in a minute his wife is with him, June Potter. She's a knockout, a splendidly beautiful woman. It takes Bairstow a moment to recover, the breath having been momentarily taken from him. She's a slim, dark woman who wears her long hair in a coif. Her eyes are so blue they're almost violet, and her skin is clear and luminous, as is a model's. Her body is so finely structured that it doesn't appear as if it's got any bones, like that of a ballet dancer. Bairstow remembers her voice instantly from the times he's called Potter to surgery: it's a slow, soft voice, deep in her throat, which makes one pause to take in every word. Usually Bairstow finds that kind of voice annoying because one has to put such attention on it, but in June Potter it's merely entrancing. He shakes her hand, a cool impression of slimness only, then he's shaking hands with Potter, whose hand he's rarely shaken in his life, though he's seen it before him--swapping instruments, probing, suturing, incising--more than any other hand he knows, maybe even Miriam's. It impresses Bairstow that this is an entirely separate occasion, one he has to get used to, when Potter isn't before him wearing surgical gloves.

Potter and his wife lead them into the living room; that's different, too, a sunken area surrounded by couches tossed with casual pillows. Is one really expected to go down there? Bairstow wonders: It's a little like a swimming pool without water--but he has to admit that it looks tempting and perhaps---what's the word Miriam always uses?--cozy.

The women are talking together: Bairstow can hear their voices as if in a dream, Miriam's firmer one, June's more hushed tones. Potter is asking him if he wants a drink. Bairstow nods, feeling as if he's answering in an insufficiently loud voice to be heard. "Scotch," he says finally. He walks back with Potter to the kitchen: it has a high ceiling, with copper pots hanging from an iron rack and a wok open on a wide counter. The entire place is white, like a surgery, yet Bairstow is impressed.

"You have a very nice home," Bairstow says, not able to come up with anything else. "You've been in this house long?" He can't remember what Potter has told him about this place, if anything--when he'd moved into it, for instance. Potter, Bairstow realizes instantly, as if in a revelation, is as uncommunicative as he, Bairstow, can be. Maybe it's some kind of damned professional affliction, Bairstow wonders. Why on earth don't I know more about Potter?

"Two years. We were going to build, but then we found this, because June said she wanted modern."

Potter somehow seems to be conveying something, but Bairstow can't catch it: did the man like modern or not? The sentence is open-ended, unanswered. The moment passes, like a skipped heartbeat.

Bairstow searches around for another tack. "You're off today, Jeff? Were you able to manage it without difficulty?" It's such a routine question, but Bairstow knows it implies so much: was Potter up last night with his patients so that today he feels wilted? Bairstow doesn't want to talk shop, but it's the place to begin.

Potter smiles and shakes his head. "Kulick's covering tonight until midnight. He wants to go away next week, so he's trying to log a little time."

"Good," says Bairstow. He raises his glass. He's feeling better now, more at home. Potter is preparing drinks for the women, but for a minute they're here together, man-to-man. There's a comfort, a familiarity even in this unfamiliar place, and Bairstow enjoys it.

"You found your new bike?" Bairstow asks. "You said you were looking."

Potter looks up, interested. "I'm having it made, did I tell you? A Belgian company. In my opinion, they make the best bikes going. Precision stuff. It'll take a month, six weeks maybe."

Bairstow nods: he's had an inkling that there's some sort of crisis about this, that Potter's been looking for a bike for a long while now. Maybe Potter will tell him; Bairstow doesn't feel it appropriate to ask. After all, he and Potter aren't soul mates; they merely meet on business of their peculiar, specialized sort.

The women are sitting in that absurd pit, making light conversation. Miriam, Bairstow notices, looks perfectly at ease, as if she were used to sitting submerged most of her life. But Miriam has always looked at ease in social situations for as long as Bairstow has known her, far more so than he, even though she protests her awkwardness. June has one leg crossed, her head to one side, listening attentively to something Miriam's been saying. She's wearing some kind of pajama, open at the neck, with strings of thin gold chains and gold sandals. Bairstow finds himself unable to take his eyes from her, it's as though he's having trouble with cardiac spasm. He's even holding his breath: silly, he thinks, but there it is. Trying to be casual, he follows Potter, who's leisurely leading the way down into the sunken area. Once there, he has to admit it's pretty nice: he sits beside Miriam, sinking into the cushions. She catches his eye: she's enjoying herself here. In a minute June has excused herself and returns with things to eat in little dishes, things to dip, and hot little rolls. It's too much: Potter entertains like a king, wooing him almost, or thanking him, one or the other. Bairstow intercepts the message, but feels that any thanks to be offered must be his, because Potter is such a good assistant. He relaxes with the scotch. When June leans over him to pass, he's aware of her perfume, something heavy and sultry, not like her at all. Somehow the name June fits her, she's young and looks poised on the verge of something, he can't tell what.

"How are your children?" June asks Miriam. "I understand you have two boys and a daughter."

Miriam smiles. "The boys are twins. Our daughter, Amanda, is in prep school, she started last fall." She wonders how much June knows about Amanda, but June seems merely interested.

"I wish we had children," she says, leaning forward. "Maybe the time will come. I pray it will. But for now, at least, our time is our own." Bairstow watches her as she drinks a stinger, sipping it with unconscious grace, her neck inclined forward as she listens to the talk flowing about her. He judges her to be not thirty, perhaps barely into her middle twenties, ten years Jeff's junior. Bairstow doesn't know if she's conscious that he's looking at her, but he tries not to stare, striving to keep his eyes averted, though he has trouble with it. Potter seems unaware, as does Miriam. Well, there's no harm in looking at one's hostess, is there? After all, it's only polite, and she's lovely, inviting admiration.

June leaves to prepare something in the wok, and Bairstow asks if he can watch, saying that he's thought of purchasing a wok and wants to see how all the preparation is done, he and Mirium had recently dined in a Japanese restaurant. That's true, he'd even communicated the concept to Miriam, asking if it wouldn't be easier to throw everything into one pot and cook it all at once as that chef had done, but Miriam had countered by saying that you just didn't throw everything into a pot and expect it to turn out the way it had for that chef. Yet Bairstow follows and stands watching June, fascinated, in that surgical kitchen while she heats the oil and cuts the remaining vegetables.

"You make me nervous, watching," she confesses with a smile, chopping with studied care. "I'm just learning, you see; I'm not an expert. A neighbor showed me how. So I'm experimenting on you a little. I hope you don't mind."

Bairstow thrusts his hands into his pockets, trying to appear nonchalant. "I don't mind at all. In fact, I'm flattered." There's a hypnotic quality about her hands: the simple gold wedding band and a small sapphire on her right hand flash before him. She has beautiful fingers, long and tapered: he'd like to tell her that he admires them, but it would be inappropriate. Bairstow feels that he's never entirely at ease with women, but then, are women entirely at ease with men? He wonders if his hesitancy might be because so many of his formative years were taken up with studying, but doubts it; instead he blames it on his Catholic upbringing, which taught in both subtle and overt ways that sex was sinful. Yet he feels at home here, in this kitchen with June.

"I'm so glad you came tonight," she says. "You and Mrs. Bairstow--Miriam. We so seldom entertain. Jeff doesn't particularly like having company. But he likes you. He thinks you're a very good surgeon."

Bairstow shifts a little and leans against the counter; he places his drink on the smooth surface. Now he can smell her perfume again in the still room, with only the faint hum of equipment somewhere. "We respect each other," says Bairstow. "We're a good team. You have to be suited temperamentally as well as technically to survive. Lots of surgical partnerships fall apart when they don't respect each other."

"So I understand. My father was a surgeon. He used to say the same thing."

"You came from around here? Your father practiced locally?"

"My father was chief-of-service at Mass. General. His name was Willoughby, maybe you've heard of him."

Jake Willoughby! Who in medical circles hadn't heard of Willoughby? He wrote the textbook they'd used in medical school. He'd even been their attending surgeon at rounds during fourth year.

"I can't think of anyone who doesn't know your father," says Bairstow. "He was...is...a pioneer in thoracic surgery. He has a clamp named after him, I use it occasionally myself." Why didn't Potter tell him, Bairstow wonders. A man as successful as Willoughby?

"So I'm told. Jeff showed it to me one time. He brought it home."

"Your father didn't show you what it looked like? I would have thought..."

"Yes, well...father was a very busy man. We barely saw him. Night, day, he was at the hospital." June momentarily takes her lip between her small, white teeth: it seems an unpleasant memory. Bairstow wonders what his children really think of him: do his long absences, his days and nights at the hospital, bug them, too? If they do, it can't be helped.

June has stopped talking, to look at Bairstow. "You want me to help?" he asks. "After all, I'm supposed to know something about slicing, you know." Both pause, then fall into instant laughter. Bairstow can't help it, he watches June shake her head to dispel tears, and it hits his funnybone again. He's flattered he said something so amusing, but damn, it *is* funny after all. He grasps a knife from the magnetic rack and begins to microtome the celery into tiny, dicey slices. "I knew you could do it," says June, and they're off again.

Potter and Miriam, having obviously heard their laughter, enter the kitchen. "What on earth...?" says Potter. "You've got the guests preparing the meal?" There's amusement there, too, and a faint undercurrent of wonder that his wife is so lively tonight...but maybe disapproval, too. Bairstow himself can't quite fathom it--but he feels a bond of camaraderie with June, and knows that she's felt it, too.

"My request," says Bairstow. "I've been talking too much, so it was only fair I offered to help. Why didn't you tell me, Jeff, that Willoughby was June's father? I knew him a little, a least well enough to make rounds together."

Potter shrugs. "Didn't think of it, I guess. Didn't even realize there'd be the connection."

Even when Willoughby taught at Bairstow's medical school and Potter must have known? Bairstow wonders if it's a touch of professional jealousy on Potter's part for his wife's father, one of the great leaders among healers. Bairstow's been told that doctors are among the most competitive of men, and perhaps it's true. But just surviving medical school was for him beyond competition—it was instead for Bairstow a matter of survival to overcome the exhaustion of long hours on the wards, intensive study, and little sleep. What Potter and his father-in-law experienced was beyond his understanding, but the fact still remains that Potter by marriage is in the family of a man at the pinnacle of his profession and revered by his peers. Not to mention this to Bairstow before this? Well, maybe it is a competition thing between the two men, who knew?

Potter and Miriam watch while June and Bairstow finish the slicing: it's a little bit funny still, and Miriam has a silly smile watching Bairstow who won't touch a thing at home. He says he's all thumbs. Obviously that's far from true.

"You're all invited to watch," says June. "You may just have to come to my rescue, though. I told Ben that I'm new to this business, but it's kind of fun. You just stir and keep adding ingredients. Jeff, check the French bread, please. Everything's set on the terrace."

The terrace, just off the kitchen, is a room under glass, like a greenhouse. It has a brick floor, the bricks set into an intricate, circular pattern. A high roof lets light bathe the interior from the setting sun, while indirect lights in the room just turning on make it seem suspended, untethered to the rest of the house and seemingly floating by itself with an almost incandescent gleam. Sliding doors open the interior to striking grounds tumbling with flowering plants of red, blue and lavender.

"It's beautiful," says Miriam as Jeff seats her before the table arranged with shining silver and pink linen. "This is just like sitting out under the stars."

"It was really an afterthought," says Potter, an enigmatic smile on his face. "We'd already built the rest of the house, and June said she wanted a glass room. Besides, it would trap heat, she said, like a solar home. Actually, it does."

Bairstow assists June by passing the rolls while Potter decants the wine. "I *love* it," June says. "I really do, I adore it, it's not an impersonal room to me at all. We both spend a great deal of time here. Even our dog won't give it up, sleeping here all winter in the sun so we can hardly get rid of him when we have company. He's really appropriated the place as his very own. Why, he sulks in the garage until we let him return." Her animation, Bairstow notices, brings a glow to her cheeks as she laughs at the understandable instincts of her dog, now banished to the garage once again.

"I can understand," says Miriam, laughing, too. "I'd never get anything done. I'd sit all day in the sun, too."

"You must come another time," June says to Miriam. "On a sunny day, just to see how pleasant it is. And to have lunch with me, of course."

Miriam looks up, surprised. "Why, I'd love to. It must be beautiful here by day, too."

The table is glass, and Bairstow has the feeling that his plate is sliding around in space, untethered. He's never felt quite that way before; it's a new sensation, trying to keep up with his plate as the invisible table disappears from view. Yet it's not unpleasant, it's as if he were confronted with a puzzle he knows will resolve itself eventually, and he merely notes it with pleasurable detachment. So much this evening escapes his usual range of habitual observations that he's given himself up to it, not questioning but merely accepting.

"It's absolutely delicious," says Miriam, still smiling as she samples the serving June has placed before her. "You're more of an expert than you think."

"Then I must owe it to Ben," June answers with a laugh and a toss of her head. "I've never been an expert before, have I, Jeff? I can be a terrible cook on occasion, and at best I'm merely passable."

Bairstow laughs, too. "I can't take credit, I'm afraid. In the kitchen I merely follow orders. Gourmet chefs would cry at my efforts." He's feeling particularly mellow now, from the scotch, wine and conversation, and Miriam is smiling at him again.

"Well, I bet he'd be marvelous," says June. "Maybe it's a latent talent and all he needs is a little encouragement."

Bairstow shakes his head and decides to change the subject: one evening of slicing celery is a far cry from devoting more of one's efforts to futile culinary pursuits.

Afterward, while the women pick up, he and Potter stroll outside briefly, even though the night air is brisk. "You really have a great place here," says Bairstow. "June seems so happy here. It obviously suits her."

"I dare say she loves it," says Potter. "After all, it's hers."

"You mean she owns it?"

"Yes. Her family's loaded, if you'll pardon the expression. Besides her father, her mother's a DuPont." He shakes his head, his eyes fixed on the rolling lawn beneath their feet. "I think they look on me as a poor relation."

Bairstow glances at Potter to see if he's joking. He isn't. "But you're a doctor, and a damned good one, Jeff. I don't know what you're talking about."

"But he's a big city specialist. The patent on that clamp alone brings in a good pile every year. By the way, did you realize we'd used one on that nurse, Helen Proctor, last week?"

Bairstow nods. "Believe it or not, I often use one. She's doing well--the nurse, I mean. Terrific, isn't it? She'll probably go home in a week or so. Fantastic woman."

Jeff Potter glances back at Bairstow, so that his eyes are lit in the light from the house. "I'm glad, Ben." He looks away. "But if it sounds like it, I'm not upset about this house. It's a nice house even if it *is* a showcase."

Bairstow ponders his partner's remark, understanding and not understanding at the same time. He thinks Potter's confidence may have eroded because his wife has put the roof over his head--and for all Bairstow knows, maybe June's money brings home some of the groceries, too. Perhaps it makes Potter feel as if he's working at some kind of hobby when he goes to the office every day. But, on the other hand, Bairstow doesn't think it would phase him one bit if Miriam were suddenly to hit the jackpot in a lottery; in fact, he'd revel in it. But it isn't the same thing, and Bairstow recognizes the fact. But if one had a wife like June, what would there be to complain about, anyway?

They can see the women walking past the long windows, and the men turn back. "Thanks for coming tonight," says Potter suddenly, turning toward Bairstow. "It's been nice having you...and meeting Miriam." Potter says it in such an ingenuous way that Bairstow turns to look at him. "Well...thanks, Jeff. Thanks for asking us. Frankly, we don't go out that often. You've been kind to us and we'd like to have you come to see us, too."

Potter seems to be considering Bairstow's words, pondering them somehow in his precise mind. "That would be nice," he says after a moment. "June would like that, too. She seemed to take to both of you immediately."

They rejoin the women. All are standing now; June hands Potter and Bairstow slim cups of cappuccino, topped with cream and shaved chocolate, which the women are already enjoying. June seems now not as tall as Bairstow had thought on first meeting her: her head rises barely beyond his chin--he can see the silver clasp holding her hair. Miriam, though, is shorter yet. She has broadened over the hips during the last years but it barely shows: after all, women are supposed to widen after children are born. June, Bairstow notices, is almost too thin by contrast: the pajamas she is wearing have hidden her body earlier, but now, standing with an arm close to her hip, he can see the material pressed against her waist and breast, making her appear lean as a child. Her face, with the thinness, is particularly fine-boned and delicate, almost like Amanda when she was a young teenager. What they'd gone through with Amanda!, he thinks inadvertently, the memory burning briefly, but then he pushes the thought away. He doesn't want to dwell on it right now, here, tonight.

"Tell me more about your children," says June, looking at Bairstow and allowing the material about her body to release at the same time. "Jeff seems to have told me, but..." She looks apologetic, as if she's made a breach of manners, but Miriam smiles. "Our boys are only twelve, not quite teenagers. *Then*, I suppose, they'll lead us a merry chase. And our daughter...seems to be enjoying school. But time will tell, this is her first semester."

"Oh, yes," says June. Now she remembers, Bairstow prepares for it. The one arrested for shoplifting, June must be thinking, what a shame. He's used to the expression by now, because everyone knows, it's even been in the court records of the newspaper.

But June appears saddened by what she appears to remember and her eyelids flicker ever so slightly. "It must be difficult when one of your children is away--I'm sure they are missed. Yet, it must give you a chance for other activities. I fill my spaces with painting, especially when Jeff is away racing on weekends."

"How wonderful," answers Miriam. "I wish I had a talent as you do, it would give me something to do all the time Bairstow's gone. The twins are so self-sufficient now. I seem to merely putter, losing valuable time...from something, I don't even know what."

When she says it, the others smile: it's said in such a winsome, off-hand way, not merely in an attempt to be merely conversational. Yet it isn't a dour comment: Miriam's chagrin seems ephemeral, as if she's really fully in charge of her free time. When Bairstow protests, on the verge of laughter, "But, Mimi, you *do* keep busy," she flushes and laughs herself. "I'm trying to fill time, to make it productive," she says finally.

It seems unusual to Bairstow, and somehow miraculous that the circles of all their separate lives have somehow had a chance to overlap, or at least to touch one another, this evening. They stand on the elevation above the sunken living room looking down into the well--and Bairstow suddenly feels as if he's miraculously conquered the feeling that he'll step back into the moat, toppling head over heels. He wonders if Potter ever has. Tonight Bairstow seems to be flying, soaring over the space like a sharp-eyed hawk, or even an eagle, coursing deftly through the space and looking down from a certain wise but distant detachment. It's a feeling he's seldom had before, but he revels in it.

"Well, perhaps we'd better leave," says Miriam finally. She's the leave-taker; Bairstow has always known that she'd exit at the proper time, that she has the social instinct for it. Yet, for once, he'd as soon stay. But Miriam has her hand extended to Potter, who's standing closest.

"It's been such a pleasure, getting to know you," she says. "Ben talks about you all the time, Jeff, saying that you're his good right arm. I don't know what he'd do without you." It isn't entirely true, Bairstow reflects, but it *is* true that Potter's getting better, a little more valuable every day, and this week with that nurse was exceptional.

"I'm flattered," says Potter, suddenly surprised. "Needless to say, the feeling is mutual. But you already know that, Bairstow."

Bairstow doesn't know it, he's wondered how Potter felt about him on more than one occasion...and it's nice to know, to have the man put it into words.

For once June appears momentarily non-plussed, as if the correct words, or the ones she'd wanted to say, fail her. "Please come again," she says. "Both of you. It's been a really, well, marvelous evening."

The Bairstows depart in the Lexus. "Did you enjoy yourself, Mimi?" Bairstow asks. "You seemed to, anyway."

"So did you, Bairstow. I can't think when I've seen you so...relaxed and alive. You don't like social gatherings."

"I know. This one was different. They're nice people. Let's make sure we see them again."

"Let's," she answers with feeling. "I'd really like that."

CHAPTER FIVE

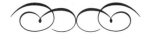

Next day, the two men, Potter and Bairstow, are in surgery again. The patient is a former teacher of Monica Levine, who just happens to have been scheduled to assist that day, having replaced Peggy Hagerty who has the flu. Neither man has as yet mentioned the evening at Potter's: business before socializing, it's always been Bairstow's credo. Their attention is riveted on the case before them though, despite his attempts, memories of June flash in on him--her hands, her smile--and he has to acknowledge that the night spent with the Potters was for him one of the nicest times he's experienced in recent memory.

Charlotte Kirkham is the head nurse today as she was with the patient Helen Proctor. Bairstow likes Charlotte to assist in his cases because she's capable and unflappable; she's been in the business long enough so she feels at home. Unfortunately, she likes to joke during surgery, but Bairstow doesn't really mind even if most of her jokes are terrible. "You hear the one about the rich old guy who asks the young girl to marry him? 'What about sex?' she asks. 'In-frequently,' he answers. 'Is that one word or two?' the girl asks doubtfully." Bairstow chuckles dutifully; it isn't very funny but he doesn't want to flatten Charlotte. The case is in the preliminary stages, nothing's happened to cause concern, it's all right to joke.

Monica's teacher is a mild, gray-haired man not yet sixty. He's trim, in very good condition, and even had a few words with Monica before he was sedated, before Ferraro put him under. His X-ray hangs in a light box behind the operating room table where Bairstow can see it. The implied malice of that film will be revealed only when Bairstow discovers in finite detail more about the shadow, precisely where it is in exact location to other organs. Yesterday Bairstow had returned to the hospital at night to study the film, then went upstairs to talk to the man. Bairstow could see the man's hands shaking as they discussed those films.

"It's definitely a tumor, Mr. Weldon, in the lower bowel, about 11 inches above the anus. All I can tell you is that the X-ray looks promising because the tumor is small and easy to remove. We can incise six inches or so of intestine on either side of it and join the remaining bowel together--that way you'll still have a colon, but it'll be a little shorter. If things are as they appear to be, you'll have no colostomy. And you'll never miss that section. I'd say the prognosis is very good."

Bairstow knows that his patients are scared to death when he mentions surgery, but he can't help it. There's no way he knows of to ease the shock or pain or fear. Sometimes, he thinks, *I'm fearful, too; I don't want to see what's in there.* These people who entrust their bodies to me are real, live people, and I'll see them after surgery, to look them in the eye and try to guide their lives thereafter. He feels skill and judgment to be very real commodities, not abstract virtues one engraves on a plaque hanging on an office wall. Yet he frequently agonizes over his decisions. He's reminded of one of Kulick's jokes: "A general practitioner, an internist and a surgeon go duck hunting. They make a bet--the other two have to buy dinner for the man who gets the first duck, but if any of the three shoot a bird who isn't a duck, he pays the other two a hundred bucks each. A flock of birds flies over, and the men aim their guns. The general practitioner shoots the first bird, saying, 'There's a bird, it sure looks like a duck.' The internist says, 'There's a bird, it looks like a duck, on the other hand it might not be. Of course,there's the off chance that it might be a...' The bird meanwhile flies away. The surgeon says, 'There's a bird'...and fires. Afterward, he adds, 'God, I sure hope that was a duck.'"

But Bairstow's never worried that he shoots too fast, because, like the internist, he agonizes too much. But he takes pains to be sure it's a duck before he shoots. This time, on Weldon, he's not entirely sure what that shadow means, but there's no other hope but to delve in and find out. It's a calculated risk; it can't be delayed too long while one inquires into the genus of the bird.

Yesterday he'd been thinking of June when he drove home, remembering the shape of her neck, the way they'd prepared the ingredients for the wok, the way they'd laughed together. She had appeared so childlike in some ways, so womanly in others, so slim and elfin. He'd thought of her hands again: the long tapered fingers, high cuticles, nails painted a pale, iridescent pink. Not a child's hands, certainly, but not quite a woman's, either. Something had touched him profoundly about her at Potter's, in a way a woman hadn't touched him in years, and today's he's decided what it was, in a fleeting revelation even as he's trying to push all extraneous thoughts away: her vulnerability. She's a vulnerable, fascinating woman: shy, gentle...but he knows as surely as he's standing in the operating room that he'll see her soon again, he simply knows the fact. It's eerie, unscientific and unprovable, but he knows it nonetheless. Confident of his knowledge, he lets it slide from his mind.

Bairstow wonders why this patient, Weldon, had been so shaken when he'd been informed that the prognosis was *good*. Bairstow can't understand it: if the prognosis had been bad, it would have made more sense. The man had begun to shake and moan, so that at first Bairstow had thought he'd not heard the optimistic words. But when he repeated them, Weldon had carried on even more, until Bairstow had considered having the man hospitalized. Miraculously, the man's derangement had cleared, and he'd insisted upon being put on the schedule at the earliest opportunity. Most people are stoics when facing their surgery, but Weldon, who'd been a self-controlled man all his life, according to Monica, had let his feelings flow all at once. He'd not even remembered the episode later when Bairstow alluded to it. It was awesome, Bairstow had thought, the capabilities of the mind, and the unexpected turns and twists that fabulous organ was capable of.

After an hour, Bairstow has dissected down to the site of the man's X-ray shadow. He holds the loop of gut harboring the tumor and feels carefully about it. It moves, flexible, without adhesions to another organ. "It looks favorable from this aspect," he tells Potter, who's holding the organs apart so he can have an unfettered look. "It's easy to mobilize, see? No attachments of any kind."

"Good sign," says Potter in a matter-of-fact voice.

They're back again to the relationship they've had for so long now: professional, impersonal, supportive within bounds. If Bairstow goofs, the mistake is on Bairstow's head alone; that's the way it has to be. If Potter makes a mistake, it's still on Bairstow's head because he's the surgeon-in-chief.

Bairstow reaches up under the intestines and feels the lobes of the liver, where bowel cancer usually migrates, where he might still find a surprise waiting. He ranges over the liver with his fingers, and as he's probing here and there he catches Monica's worried look, and he knows that she's wondering what the difficulty is with her teacher, almost fearing what Bairstow's fingers will uncover. She seems to be holding her breath. "Relax, Monica," he says, "I don't feel any metastases in the left lobe...and, no, none in the right lobe, either."

He can see Monica's eyes over the mask: they narrow and lengthen, and Bairstow can tell she's smiling. It's nice, he thinks, to have made someone happy for once. Potter relaxes, too, as does Charlotte Kirkham. Everything's on an even keel now, almost routine, except that there's nothing routine in surgery. Bairstow knows it in his bones. Yet now they come as close to feeling jubilant in the operating room as they ever do. The cleaned end of the severed gut, clamped off half an inch back by duck-billed hemostats, looks fat and healthy. Monica leans forward to clamp a bleeder. "Good work, Monica," says Bairstow. "You're right on the ball."

Bairstow is exerting effort all the time, and discipline; yet the thought of June's silver hair clasp enters his head unbidden. He glances at Potter, bent forward and working intently to close, and tries to shove the thought from his mind. He tries to put his entire attention on sewing with the curved needles in their long-handled holders. The surgical field is wide before him, the patient opened diagonally in from the navel, below and between the iliac arch and down into the funnel inside the pelvic cradle. Bairstow can feel his own rhythmic motion as he stitches, moving his hips slightly beneath the surgical gown, testing then retesting the stitches, pulling tight, slackening, then pulling tight again. It's a kind of rhythm he's used to; it feels good, efficient, smooth. A latticework of clamps holds the tissue as he stitches. He summons Monica briefly to his side, then hands her the severed gut containing the tumor to send to pathology for verification of its composition, then inserts the colon stapler, resembling a caulking gun, into Weldon's anus. He knows this man, Weldon, but now he tries to think of him distantly as he suffers him these indignities—he's glad Weldon can't look him in the eye and tell him to go to hell. He slides the free end of the man's colon down into the machine's tip from the inside, then fires a ring of stainless steel staples into it. As a last measure, he dumps a gallon of warm saline into the wound. No bubbles, says Potter, bending to examine as if he might be inspecting a leaky tire: air isn't escaping or entering, the seal is holding tight

Bairstow closes, then sutures the incision with monofilament. Job done, tumor successfully removed.. Now the man can become Weldon again, he can resume personhood.

"That was a nice dinner Saturday night," says Bairstow to Potter. They're taking turns in the shower again, removing the sweat and blood acquired during the course of the last two hours of work.

"We enjoyed having you, Ben. June thought you and Miriam were both terrific. She wants you to come again."

"Our turn next. Except that our house isn't as impressive." Bairstow knows he's speaking truthfully, that their old Victorian place rambles all over the lot. But in no way, he reflects, could he tolerate Potter's sunken living room for long.

"Sounds great," says Potter. "After the bike season. Coming up pretty fast now."

Unbidden, Bairstow's heart sags a little: he'd thought he might have seen June much sooner than that. The way Potter said it, it sounds as if the bike season lasts months and months of weekends.

Somewhat depressed, Bairstow heads to his office, to face the day. His appointment book is solid, says Val Hobson, his appointment secretary, looking at him just a little reproachfully because he's already goofed up her afternoon by arriving a half-hour late from surgery and jamming up the early patients already waiting for him. The list she's placed on his desk is so long that he doesn't even have a chance to look it over. He dons his white coat and finishes an apple, the tailend of his lunch which had included a sandwich from the snack bar. But he's not particularly hungry because a successful surgery always leaves him stimulated and he can't eat when he's aroused with happy excitement.

First on his appointment is a professor from a law school, referred by his local physician. The poor man has been battling cancer for five years. Five years ago other surgeons took out a perforated colon, riddled with cancer, then later removed more and more. Heroic surgery, to save a life. The man has been continuing to teach law students even with all that going on, but now he's had a recurrence and Bairstow knows he's helpless to do a damn thing.

In the next examining room, says Jan Valenti, his nurse, is a plastics engineer who's contracted a rare bile-duct cancer. Bairstow wonders if it's job-related in any way--lots of cancers he sees are. He can tell when he opens a patient whether he or she smokes, lives on a dusty road, or endures a city's pollution by examining the black residue in the alveoli of the lungs. He once had a man who worked for a major cigarette company tell him that smoking was much exaggerated as a cause of disease. Bairstow had grasped him about the biceps, virtually lifting him from the examining table, instructed him to dress, then showed him the door. "If you should ever change jobs and philosophies, I'm here," Bairstow told the man. "Until then, find another doctor." Bairstow feels that he hasn't been involved with patients trying desperately to get well all these years to have to suffer idiots who spread the disease he's pitted against.

In the third room, Jan says, indicating the chart in her hand, is a schoolteacher with stomach cancer. Bairstow shakes his head: this woman knows what's going on, too. Her internist has sent her to him thinking she has a stomach ulcer, but the woman has said all along she thought it wasn't an ulcer at all.

"Does she have a chance?" Jan asks compassionately. Bairstow knows that Jan, being young and inexperienced, has replaced another nurse who left the area to marry and is going to take a while to adjust to the realities of a day-in, day-out medical practice, but today is especially tough on her. He goes home some nights with his own stomach knotting from some of the somber diagnoses of patients he's seen that day.

Bairstow takes the chart from Jan's hand and reviews it briefly. "About zero," he says, at least that's what the long-term studies show. "But lately we've been hearing about some new forms of chemotherapy that seem to help more than the old ones. We'll give it a try, Jan. Don't look so dejected."

"But it's so *awful*. And won't chemotherapy make her terribly sick?"

Bairstow nods. "I'm afraid so, but there's no way around it, at least at the present time. We've got limited tools, but we're gaining. Maybe it helps to look at it that way."

"All right, Dr. Bairstow, I'll...try."

"Who's in my office, Jan?"

"Terry Levine, the boy with Hodgkin's disease." But her face is still so crestfallen that Bairstow turns back to her. "Jan, you've got to figure that many of the people here will live. We're not to blame for their illnesses; we help all we can even if we can't cure them now. Look at it like this--we keep them alive a little longer, have ways of making them more comfortable, and maybe in the added time a cure will come along." He pauses a moment. "I wish we were God, but we aren't. Being merely mortal, we do the best we can."

Jan looks down at the charts in her hand. "I'm sorry, Dr. Bairstow. I'm a nurse and I should be used to this by now. I'll try."

"The truth is it isn't easy for any of us, Jan." They walk together into Bairstow's office, a moderately large room with a view out onto the hospital lawn. He shares this area of the building with an internist, a proctologist, and an ENT specialist. He's rented for twelve years now, since the building was erected, and hasn't moved since. He feels comfortable here and would hate to leave.

Waiting before his desk is a giant of a teenager, a mammoth young man wearing pants with suspenders, an old shirt and worn, bespattered shoes.

"Sit down," says Bairstow. "How are you, Terry?" He sizes the boy up: he's pale, apprehensive. "Do you remember Miss Valenti here?"

The boy raises his hand briefly. "How'ya?" he says, going through the gestures, not really caring.

"How's the truck-driving business?" Bairstow asks with a smile, trying to put him at ease but not succeeding.

"Okay, it's okay." He sits down reluctantly.

"He has growths on his neck," explains Jan, anxious to get away from her insecurities and into her professional role. "I examined him when he arrived, Dr. Bairstow. On the left side, you see here." Jan indicates the surface in question.

Bairstow slides forward on his office chair and feels the boy's neck where Jan has indicated, though the lumps are plainly visible without touching them. Bairstow's fingers trace the outline of the tumors, like rocks or barnacles on a piling. "Remember, I told you last time," Bairstow says, "that you might have Hodgkin's disease, that I thought it a possibility? We took a series of tests?"

The boy nods, not looking at Bairstow.

"Well, we've confirmed that diagnosis. It *is* Hodgkin's, Terry. I wish I could tell you otherwise. But 85 percent of all people who get it can be cured completely. The chances are very good that we can help you. Please don't look so depressed. We really can, with X-rays and medicine."

Just then the phone interrupts, at a bad time, with the boy before him suffering agonies. He looks into the outer office and sees that Val is not at her desk. Bairstow finds himself talking to someone in the records office, who tells him his charts aren't complete, that unless they're finished by six o'clock the hospital will withdraw operating privileges. It's the old story, the hospital administration is again acting like the hostile bureaucracy it is. "I'll get there," says Bairstow, thoroughly exasperated. "Don't call me, I'll call you." He wonders again whether, if he were to become chief of the surgical service as has been rumored, he could accomplish anything because the bureauocracy is so entrenched. It's already a hard day, and the administration of his own hospital has only made it worse. He takes the phone off the hook and leaves it there, not wanting to be interrupted again.

Terry Levine is staring out Bairstow's window without twitching a muscle. Jan Valenti has disappeared into the waiting room to check another patient. "We'll need to take a bit of tissue from your neck," Bairstow begins again, as if in continuing conversation, "and from the hard gland beneath your arm, Terry. Then we'll know more what we're talking about."

The boy stares at Bairstow, not moving a muscle, not flinching.

Bairstow persists, trying to elicit a response from the boy, any response; he appears in psychological shock. "I think your cancer is treatable, Terry--do you hear me?--cancer of the lymph glands. We need to have you in the hospital for a biopsy. Miss Valenti can schedule it for you. Am I getting through to you?"

The boy stands; for a moment, he doesn't say a word. "Okay," he says, his voice muted. "I hear you." He turns to go. "You want me to leave this door open or closed?"

Even Bairstow is shaken this time: won't the boy say anything more? Won't he vent his frustration some way, even by slamming the door?

Bairstow has a momentary impulse to run after him and try again to help him face his problem. But then he decides instead to call him on the phone after Terry has a chance to assimilate the information, when the initial shock has passed and the boy realizes that Bairstow has said it's a treatable, curable disease.

Bairstow sits down at his desk, agonizing about what to write on the boy's chart. Has the young man no emotion left, so hard is the shock? Is he emotionally unstable? How would Terry have reacted if the outlook were truly bleak? But Bairstow has a sudden, jarring thought: how would *he* react if he had been told that cancer had invaded his own body, that it was eating relentlessly at his own tissues, even if the prognosis was ultimately hopeful? Would he still deny it as the boy had done? Bairstow has known colleagues who wouldn't tell a soul when they themselves contracted a fatal disease, and still others who spoke of it freely. What would he himself do, Bairstow wonders, after the first 10 pounds of weight loss, 15, 20? He turns back to his chart: such thoughts get him nowhere, after all, when he has work to do. He must shed the anxiety about the boy, for he will undoubtedly come in for treatment and get cured. And, yes, he'd probably have acted like his colleague, keeping his own counsel about his private condition: what good would it do to rail against fate, over which one has no control?

Bairstow strides into the office where the law professor waits. The man's reading a book, a small paper backed volume entitled *Current Problems in Corporate Law*. The man's thinner, grayer, more stooped, but smiling, alive, full of enthusiasm for his circumstances, as if nothing were wrong. As if, Bairstow thinks, he's made a private bargain with death.

"How are you doing?" asks Bairstow kindly--he enjoys this man, a witty, intelligent person. They chat amiably while Bairstow examines him.

"Very well, actually. I work part-time."

"Terrific. Any discomfort?"

"A little. I ignore it--otherwise I take those pills."

"I hope you're taking vacations, Mr. Schuster. You wanted to visit Russia, to review the legal system there, as I remember."

"Yes, I just may do it, but I'm so busy, you see. My students..."

The man's plucky. He carries on, he's a fighter. Bairstow's always admired pluck—many of his patients have it, perhaps the majority, and it awes Bairstow at the courage they show at the brink, as if thumbing their noses at whatever lurks on the other side.

"Well," says Bairstow, "call me if you wish, at any time, just to chat or when you need some more of those pills."

"Thank you," says the lawyer with a nod. "I intend to cheat the grim reaper for quite a few more years."

"You'll do it, too," laughs Bairstow, and walks him to the door.

"He's a fine man," Bairstow says to Jan when the professor has gone. "I admire him. I've never heard him complain, and he's got every right to. He accepts responsibility for his life, and is interested in everything."

"I'm afraid I'd complain all the time," says Jan, looking doubtful. "I'm a sissy about some things--and health is one. Perhaps that's why I wanted to become a nurse...and to help others, of course."

Bairstow smiles at her. "You probably have more courage than you know, Jan. Maybe we all do, when we're up against it."

Two hours later the waiting room is clearing. The teacher with the stomach ulcer has come and gone, and a fireman, and a farmer kicked by a bull ("The flesh will heal itself," says Bairstow, trying to conceal his smile, "but I'd advise you to curb that bull"). He glances at his list of appointments which Val Hobson has so neatly compiled, and finds another name which she's penciled in: June Potter. He can't believe it. What is June doing here?

"That lady called a little while ago," says Val, having entered the office between Bairstow's patients to see how the appointments are going. "She sounded uncertain, but I put her on the list anyway."

It seemed so miraculous--Bairstow had thought he must wait weeks, months even, to see her again, and here she is, in his waiting room. Why, he wonders. What possibly could lead her here? The same feeling overcomes him again as at the dinner: awe, quickening interest...and surprise at his own reactions. "Send her in, Val, will you please?"

CHAPTER SIX

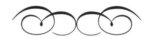

He rises and comes to the front of his desk--and then June is there. "Mrs. Potter," says Val.

"Come in, June."

She extends her hand and Bairstow clasps it. He closes the door behind her. "It's so nice to see you again. I...we enjoyed being at your house. You...and Jeff were so good to us." He feels as if he's babbling, but doesn't seem able to help it.

"We enjoyed it, too, Ben. I loved meeting you both."

Bairstow looks at her more closely now...as he is used to doing in this room. She still looks like a child. Today she has another clip on her hair, this one ivory, intricately carved, which glows in the mass of her dark hair. She is wearing an emerald green suit, closely fitted to her figure, with a bright scarf at the neck. Usually it's Bairstow's failing that he doesn't remember what his patients are wearing, but he has a vivid image of June sitting before him, looking at him as if a little reluctant to start.

"It's just that I'm short-of-breath so much of the time," she begins after a moment, her voice even lower than usual. "I don't know what it is. Probably I'm not in very good shape: I don't jog or do any of the things that Jeff does to take care of himself, and I have trouble when I walk, or when I move around very much. I'm sure you didn't notice the other night, Ben. I used to play tennis with some of my friends, but I've had to give it up, to make excuses instead. I'm...more than a little worried."

She looks at Bairstow, her eyes wide, and Bairstow knows from long experience what that look means: she's terrified, but she doesn't want to show it. She's fighting for control, and at the same time trying to convey her concern without flinching.

"What does Potter say?" Bairstow asks. "You've told him, of course."

To his surprise she shakes her head and looks down into her hands. "I...didn't want to, you see. He's so, well, involved, and maybe this is nothing. Besides, he thinks I'm a bit of a hypochondriac, and maybe he's right about that. I seem to always have complaints, and I don't do lots of things well. Somehow you encouraged me the other night, Ben...even to doing something as silly as prepare dinner. I haven't done it for ages, we haven't had company. But it was nice of you."

Bairstow sits back and looks at her appraisingly. Her skin is pale, but perhaps she's genetically fair-skinned. It's more difficult to tell obvious signs with fair-skinned people. "Do you have any pain?" he asks her, as he has with so many of his patients this day.

She thinks a moment, then shakes her head. "Something in my chest, but I can't tell. It's just this short-of-breath thing." She clasps her hands tightly together. "I'm afraid it might be something...serious, Ben, and I'm frightened. I'm trying to do as best I can...which isn't very good at the moment, I'm afraid."

Clearly, Bairstow feels, he has to do something. He wants to help, but momentarily he isn't sure where to start, especially when Potter doesn't even know of June's distress. He dismisses immediately that it's her imagination, June is too self-possessed and well-balanced for that.

He buzzes for Jan. "I'm going to examine you, June, to see if I can find anything. Jan will help you get undressed." For the first time in years Bairstow feels professionally unsure: he wants to find something in the woman's body to help explain her symptoms, yet at the same time he passionately hopes there's nothing there.

Bairstow sees another patient while waiting for June to be ready, a man whose hernia he'd repaired a month before. The man is almost healed. Bairstow examines for tenderness, and the man barely moves under Bairstow's probing. "You're doing well," Bairstow says, trying to wrench his mind from June. "Have you had any more discomfort?"

The man, a burly fellow who owns a butcher shop, shakes his head. "Nuthin' like before, Doc Bairstow. Can I go back to bowlin' soon?"

"Another week. The Lord needs a chance to make you whole, my friend. He's entitled to His say, you know."

The man sits up, his prodding over. "Hope this never happens again, Doc."

"I doubt it ever will, Henry. I want to see you soon for your last check-up, and then you're on your own."

Jan enters the room to indicate that June is ready, then stands beside the door to let Bairstow know she's available if he needs her. June is wrapped in one of the blue robes Bairstow provides for his patients. Gently he moves aside the flimsy cloth. Bairstow is overwhelmed by June's frailty; she hasn't an extra pound of flesh to shield her bones anywhere on her body, yet she is not emaciated. She has no weight at all, Bairstow feels; one could lift her like a leaf. He almost feels that he might hurt her when he examines her, so he proceeds as gently as he can.

"Show me where you think you might feel something," says Bairstow. When she indicates a place over her lung, Bairstow percusses it, trying to ferret out the hollow echoing spaces in her chest cavity.

"I can't hear a thing, June," he says after a minute. "Nothing at all. I'll see if I can pick up anything by stethoscope."

He bends to his task, roving the stethoscope over the area where she's felt the pain, then over the space occupied by the other lung. He feels an intensity about this search for the difficulty she's experiencing, hoping it's nothing more than an innocuous, persistent bronchitis or hay fever which may already have dissipated. Her heart has a clear, strong beat. He can palpate the organs of her body, which seem normal in size and elicit no pain on percussion. She has a small appendix scar but doubts if adhesions ever caused problems, and certainly not this one. He can find nothing.

"Please dress and come into my office," he says. "We'll see where we go from here."

He waits for her to come in, opening the fresh parchment of her chart, which Val has just placed on his desk with June's name neatly typed in. June Potter, it reads, the name underlined; he's pleased that she's come to him, he'll do his level best for her. He's barely begun to write on the first page when June is before him, waiting expectantly.

"Please sit down, June," he says, wishing he were on the other side of that formidable desk to seat her. He sits down himself, placing his hands on the desk before him. "I didn't find anything, but for the life of me, I don't know if that's good or bad."

He sees the relief as well as the puzzlement on her face, but presses on. "I think you should have other tests, because my examination doesn't mean much without them: X-ray, EKG, a blood profile. Would you like me to make the appointments?"

"Thanks, Ben, but I hate to take your time..."

"But I'm more than happy..." He picks up the phone: usually he leaves this to Val, but June is Potter's wife...and a friend. He feels responsible for her in some way he's just becoming aware of, but it may be because he's never had a partner's wife as a patient before.

"Val, set up an X-ray, EKG, and a profile for Mrs. Potter, will you? Let me know when they're scheduled. Mrs. Potter will be here a few minutes longer."

Bairstow has only one more patient today, and she's late although she's waiting now. Well, she'll just have to wait a little longer. "If there's anything I can do for you, I will, June. Come and see me after you have the tests at the hospital, will you? Or before, anytime. You're sure you don't want me to discuss this with Potter?"

She shakes her head. "I'll tell him myself when it's over, Ben, when the results are in." She smiles hopefully across the desk at Bairstow. "Maybe there won't be anything to tell him."

"I hope not. I'll talk the tests over with you after they're completed, to explain them to you."

"I'd appreciate that, when it's convenient for you. I'm not all that busy. My painting doesn't exactly consume all my time."

"You're a portrait painter? I wondered." Bairstow can remember the painting of a man, perhaps a younger Potter, above the fireplace in that sunken living room.

"Yes, and I do studies in still life. Water colors, too, but now I work mostly in oils."

Bairstow is impressed: he'd signed up for a painting class once long ago when he'd had more time, and had enjoyed it, but felt his talent to be incredibly thin.

Val comes back into the room, a slip of paper in her hand. "You've been scheduled for tomorrow morning, Mrs. Potter. Apparently they've had a cancellation or two. Is that convenient?"

June nods gratefully. "That's so prompt, I never expected it. You're sure you want me to come here afterward?" She looks fully at Bairstow and he's reminded again of her violet eyes.

"Of course. I have no surgery in the morning, so I should be able to review the X-rays. Give Mrs. Potter my first appointment, Val."

"Yes, sir." She hands June the slip of paper with the times of her appointments written on it, then leaves the room. June slips it into her purse, then stands. Again she extends her hand to Bairstow, and he has the instant wish to hold it, to cradle it between his larger ones. He can feel its slimness again, the fine bones so delicate that one can almost crack them if he were to squeeze too hard. "Until tomorrow then, Ben. Thanks for...facilitating things for me."

"I'm happy to, June."

She starts to leave, then turns back. "I feel comfortable with you, that's why I'm here. You're a nice person, Ben. I trust you. I'll do whatever you say, if there's trouble. I want you to know that."

Bairstow is overcome with a barrage of things he'd like to say to her; instead, he leaves his desk and holds open the door. Words seem difficult to him at this moment, as they've always been at crucial times in his life. He wishes he could say the words he wants to say, to convey how he feels, but he's not very good at it and never has been. Yet she seems to understand that; she looks at him and smiles as she walks by, leaving behind a fleeting trace of perfume.

He returns to his desk, sits behind it, pondering: on examination there was nothing, really no pathology he could find to explain her symptoms. Her shortness of breath is recent, its onset short weeks ago. She's a young woman, unathletic by her own testimonial, but even inactive young women don't usually have shortness of breath. And maybe there *had* been something in the right upper quadrant, he couldn't be sure of that. But if she is going to have X-rays tomorrow, and all the blood work, why is he sitting here worrying today? The tests may find out far better than he can what her body is hiding from his searching fingers.

He rings for Jan Valenti. "Show in the last patient, Jan, I'm ready now." He's glad the day is almost over.

Afterward, he drives home slowly, playing soft music on his CD: no medical education talks today. He has to let his mind clear. Maybe, he thinks as he has occasionally in the past at low moments, I'll leave this business someday. He reviews all the things he could have chosen instead of surgery: the Air Corps: he'd started flight training, but then the war was over. Teaching: he'd been a whiz at microbiology and even tutored other students. Or radiology: he'd admired his chief-of-service, and then he'd have fewer weekend hours. Bairstow had even gone to inquire about a residency in pediatrics and been told one might be available after he'd completed surgical rotation. A joy, he'd thought, working with young bodies for a change.

Then one night they'd brought into the hospital a policeman who'd been stabbed with a broken bottle in the temporal artery. Bairstow can still remember the horror of it: blood spurting from the man's head like a blown hose. No one there for the first few minutes had exhibited any damned sense at all, he thinks, recalling the scene vividly now as he snakes his car through the traffic. They didn't even put pressure on the bleeding wound. Within moments Bairstow had been right there in the thick of the action on the surgical emergency team covering the accident room that night. As he drives he can still feel the excitement and hear the family's screams as the cop was rushed into the hospital and down the hall.

But as Bairstow and his team had worked on the man in the emergency room, he could hear the voice of a pediatrician on call talking on the wall phone behind him with even-tempered forbearance to a patient: "Mrs. Jessup, all you have to do is boil the milk a little longer, then the baby won't vomit so often." Bairstow, trying to stanch the man's blood, working against the clock, had thought: is *that* what a pediatric practice is all about, boiling milk and preparing formula? *That's* an emergency?

He'd never considered a pediatrics specialty again, because surgery was so much more fascinating to him, more real and vital. The cop had recovered quickly, Bairstow remembers, because the whole thing had appeared much worse than it seemed on first appraisal. As soon as someone applied pressure to the wound and snaked in an intravenous line, bleeding came under control quickly and the wound was routinely repaired.

At home, the twins are out in the yard working on their bicycles, Pete adjusting the spokes and Norman applying lubricant from a tube to the shifting mechanism. Bairstow remembers only too well his own fascination with engines and moving car parts and wonders if they're exhibiting early mechanical talents. They are not identical twins--Pete is a little chunkier and Norman is taller--and Bairstow acknowledges this fact with gratitude because few people have difficulty telling them apart.

"Hi," says Bairstow, looking down at the bike. "Don't you guys think it's about time to cut the lawn? Look at it, it's like a hayfield."

Pete gets off his haunches. "Come on, Dad, it isn't that bad. Norman cut it last week...or was it two weeks ago?"

"Well, we've had a lot of rain, and it's growing a foot a day. I want it cut by the weekend, okay? Look over at Mathewson's, it's a showcase. Matt's going to start complaining."

Norman is still sitting on the tarmac at the edge of the driveway. "But his is *always* perfect, Dad. Shit, he cuts it twice a week even when it doesn't need it."

Bairstow realizes the truth of Norman's words, but feels the need to exert his paternal authority, to maintain discipline. "Listen, stop swearing, all right? And when I say I want it cut, that's that. Allowances can stop pretty fast, you know." He hopes Norman hasn't noticed that he swears sometimes, too, especially in tight, emotional moments, but he feels his kids should respect his authority and not challenge his edicts. Generally they're good kids and he's proud of them. He doesn't really care what his kids say about him after they've grown up, he's thought at philosophical moments, except to recall that he'd *tried* to be a good father, and that he was fair. He has no idea what happened to Amanda to make her steal, except that her psychologist avowed during an interview with them that it was a plea for attention. "From us?" Bairstow had asked. "I don't know, Dr. Bairstow," the psychologist had answered, "that remains to be seen." Bairstow had thought: What does he mean by that?? Are we not giving her enough attention? He got very little attention as a boy, but he'd never stolen. Why, he'd wondered, don't these people say what they mean instead of laying guilt on you and being so damned enigmatic? But he had to admit that Amanda seemed a little more relaxed after talking to the man.

The twins are still looking at him. He glances at the shift on Pete's bike. "Say, that looks pretty good, Pete, neat job." He knows it comes off partly as a palliative, but he *is* proud of the way they keep up their bikes, so they can transport themselves about the city on errands, and can tend lawns and do odd jobs during the summer for neighbors. "Don't expect transportation from your mother or me," he'd said. Except that on rainy days he already knows that Miriam will throw the bikes into the van and deliver both vehicle and rider neatly at their destination. He'd been known to do it, too. "But that lawn," he repeats, "no 'ifs' or 'buts'."

"Sure, Dad," says Pete with a grin. "Gotcha."

Miriam is in the kitchen. "Hi," he says, giving her a kiss. In a mirrored pan he can see that his tie is askew and that he's been running his fingers through his hair, so that it stands in peaks. It's a clear sign that he's had a tough day, and Miriam has read the signs already. "Take a drink out on the lawn," she says. "I'll join you."

He makes himself a scotch, then carries it to the lawn chair. He hooks his cellphone, his connection to the hospital, to his belt. In five minutes Mirium joins him; she's shelling peas for dinner. She sits down in a companion chair to his. "Office hours must have been rough," she says.

He has an impulse to tell her about June, but it would be unethical, and a part of him wants to keep it private. "I'll be all right, Mimi. Sorry, I'm lousy company at the moment."

"You're just shifting gears. You know, I've been thinking, Ben. Perhaps we should ask people over more often. We don't, you know. Sometimes I think we're hermits. The other night at Potter's you seemed more cheerful than I've seen you in months. It might be good for you."

"Maybe you're right."

"It's just that we don't do things together very often, do you realize? I know you've got that hellish schedule and can't get home very often, but we seem to live our separate lives. We're not getting any younger..."

Bairstow thinks about it. "It's just that last week I worked almost a hundred hours--Jan counted them up--including the time on call, and that almost rules out social..."

"I *know* that, Ben. But do you *need* to work 100 hours? What if you took charge of the surgical staff? Could you cut the time for yourself... and others? Of course, you said they'd want you to travel, to look into other surgical house procedures, but you couldn't take any more time than you're already applying to your own practice. And maybe it would reduce your hours in the end."

She's right again, Bairstow is thinking. And he knows the fault is with himself: even if he isn't weary when he returns home, he seldom wants to mix with other doctors, to talk shop all evening as doctors always do. Nor does he often want to see laymen: some are in awe, others want free advice, the rest are knowledgeable in fields he knows nothing about and cares for even less--running department stores or banks or teaching high school English. The wives either don't work at all, or are clerks or secretaries, or run charities--although more and more are entering the work force these days. Yet what Miriam says is true, he'd like to get to know some other people. One is the law school professor he'd seen today in his practice, another an officer of a European corporation, the third a physicist from a company out on Route 128. He can understand that Miriam must feel isolated sometimes, though she does have her own pursuits, as a member of the YMCA executive board and a volunteer at a child care center. They'd felt pretty good about things until Amanda got into trouble; it had done something subtle to them in their contact with other people. They should change that around, they really should.

He shakes out the paper he'd been reading. "We could ask Hal Briggs, Mimi, you've always liked him, and Vera." Hal's a local stockbroker, they'd hear about investments all night, not caring two hoots about investments, but Miriam does like Vera. Bairstow learned a long time ago that nobody wanted to hear about his surgery, either:

as a young surgeon he'd been discussing one of his first cases, a small repair of a knife wound with his hostess, when the poor woman passed out cold on her own kitchen floor. That had taught him, and thereafter he left *his* business at the hospital where it belonged. Yet Miriam, bless her, generally seems interested in his cases, and for that he's always been grateful.

Bairstow thinks again about June: tomorrow will tell. But it still touches him that she came to seek his help. As he allows that thought to circulate throughout his brain, he acknowledges that it's the nicest thing to have happened to him in a long time. He feels better, his spirits rise. Yes, Bairstow thinks, maybe I chose the right field after all.

CHAPTER SEVEN

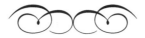

Bairstow arises early the next morning; he hadn't been able to sleep anyway. He strolls outside, still clad in his pajamas and bathrobe, but barefoot. The grass is damp with dew. He likes the early morning best because he always was a morning person, and the world seems so full of promise then. Miriam is still sleeping, her pillow tucked over her head--to shut out the world, perhaps. He walks into the greenhouse where only last week, or was it the week before, he'd determined to start gardening again. When was he going to get time to garden, anyway? It was a pipe dream. He knows very well that, despite his brief doubts of yesterday, he likes the challenge of the hospital; he responds to its vibrancy, insistent as a musical beat. Even on the seventh day, on Sunday itself, he carries along his cellphone; whether he likes it or not, he's chosen his profession, and it claims him, perhaps too much sometimes, but he'd have no other. It's a hard taskmistress, no doubt about that. He knows that, like yesterday, after an early morning respite, the rest of the day can turn relentless. He hears the slam of a window upstairs: Pete is getting up for school as is Norman in the bedroom opposite—or at least one can hope because he's heard no sound from that side of the house. Miriam will be stirring, too--she sets her alarm for seven without fail. Presently he'll see her form moving beyond the French doors.

He looks up at the old house he's provided for his family: it's a barn of a place, rebuilt and rebuilt again by subsequent owners, until he took it over. He loved its cornices and gingerbread trim as soon as the realtor showed it to him, but mostly he loved the grounds--private, replete with plantings and lovely old trees, a place where one could take a stroll, as he is this morning in his night clothes, without the world knowing. The building is certainly no architectural miracle, and the architect he'd hired to change the place around had thrown up his hands and almost refused to take the job. "We don't know what's in those walls," he'd lamented. "Maybe there's no insulation. And you know those old Victorian places, they're always full of sudden--and expensive, I might add--surprises."

Bairstow hadn't really cared what the architect thought or how much he'd complained, because Bairstow had grown up in a Victorian house, old though it was, and decrepit even in his youth, but he'd loved it just the same. Besides, there were fifty more architects in the phone book, but this man had come recommended by one of the internists, so Bairstow had called him first.

"I like this place," Bairstow had told the architect. "It's what I've always wanted, and my wife loves it, too. It's in the neighborhood I want, not far from schools, and I don't have to drive for hours to Memorial. I want that wall taken down between the living room, the parlor, and whatever that other dinky little room is called. I want it livable. I want my kids to be able to do somersaults on the living room rug just like I did when I was a kid without crashing into a wall. There's nothing wrong with that, is there?"

The architect had stopped grumbling, having received the message- and a decent advance. "But that room will be *big*, Dr. Bairstow, too damned big in my opinion. Forty-two by 38, something like that, I'll measure it. A barn of a place. Do you really want to heat it?"

"What on earth would we do with all those fussy little rooms? Sure, I'll heat it. I've always wanted a big room, anyway."

Bairstow shakes his head, remembering the conversation. The room is big, no doubt about it, but he loves it even if it costs him money to heat. He doesn't spend money on lots of extravagant treats because he doesn't have time. To diminish the size, he lined the walls with books, even his old medical tomes which he still consults on occasion, and had cabinets and closets built in on two sides. Then they found there was enough room left over for the grand piano Miriam's parents gave her. Still the room appeared large, but more in proportion than before. "At least we won't be in each other's way," he'd said philosophically to Miriam when they'd surveyed the completed area. "We'll have our own space together, and our separate areas at the same time."

"Yes," Miriam had answered with a smile, "and the children can turn somersaults without crashing into the walls." It had made Bairstow shake his head and also smile because to his knowledge, they hadn't turned a somersault in there yet.

Now it's time to go inside, he can't linger here longer with a busy day on the horizon. But it's lovely here, feeling the grass through his toes and the morning mist just beginning to dampen his bathrobe. He'd almost forgotten about that early morning surgical section meeting: one of the younger vascular surgeons, a man named Hanley, is apparently having a conflict of some kind with the ENT man. The way Bairstow understands it, the ear, nose and throat man is refusing to cover weekends for vascular emergencies even though Hanley came to town with his family after having received assurances from the surgical staff and the hospital that he'd have coverage. I'll cover him myself if necessary, Bairstow thinks. The man had come from Hawaii to set up practice here, and just because someone's decided to back down on a promise doesn't mean Bairstow will. But, of course, it's a collective matter; he'll try to resolve it as one of the senior surgeons in a way that will insure the new man's continued residence here.

Bairstow doesn't mind getting involved because Hanley, the vascular man, is young and promising and Bairstow doesn't want to lose him from the staff. When Potter is away, Hanley's even helped him in surgery on occasion. Hanley has a wife with multiple sclerosis and Bairstow feels sorry for him. In addition, the man has just lost a suit for malpractice, and Bairstow's sense of the case is that Hanley's lawyer was so incompetent, and Hanley himself so distracted by his wife's recently diagnosed problem, that it was simply an unfortunate case, a botch on Hanley's record that never should have been there. But Hanley has been letting his temper get away from him, and that will have to be considered, too.

After that, he'll have to see a few office patients, June among them. First he'll get a look at the X-rays with Ebersole, the radiologist, to see what they showed--and then later, hopefully, he can dispel her fears. When she'd seen him yesterday, her face had been set as if she were dreading his verdict. It would be nice to see her smile, Bairstow is thinking; she'd looked pinched. And maybe she was experiencing more discomfort than she'd let on, but there was no way he could divine that unless she told him--except that June appears to be the sort of person who wouldn't volunteer that information unless you pried it out of her. Bairstow understands that pride only too well, he'd seen it in other patients and done the same thing himself, refusing to confess discomfort under the mistaken notion that one should keep everything private if one could do nothing about it. Pride winning over pain, what folly! If that is June's problem, he'll have to do something about it because he doesn't want her to suffer needlessly, or to feel weak or frightened, either. Yet, he thinks, perhaps this is all unnecessary conjecture if there is nothing wrong in those X-rays: he doesn't really know June and might be jumping to conclusions. On the other hand, he spends day after day seeing one patient after another, and gets a sense of their motives and strengths and weaknesses while they confront their own mortality. Yet Bairstow shakes his head at himself as he reenters the house: this kind of introspection is uncomfortable for him. He isn't used to it, it's more exhausting than a six-hour surgical procedure. Weren't surgeons, he reminds himself again, supposed to shoot at ducks and wonder afterward what genus of fowl had been in their sights? Yet he knows he'll never be that kind of surgeon, either.

Bairstow wants only coffee this morning. He stands, reading the paper while the boys shuffle in, almost soundlessly, helping themselves to cold cereal, a morning ritual. How can they be so noisy at dinner and subdued at breakfast, he wonders idly. Miriam is already padding about the kitchen in fleece slippers because the day *is* cool although he hadn't felt it on the grass. Miriam is usually the one who prefers bare feet if there's any warmth in the air; he'd always thought of his wife as basically a child of nature tamed to indoor living only reluctantly... until recently, when she seems to have gravitated to fleece slippers and quilted robes.

Peter looks up from the kitchen table suddenly, sleep glazing his face. "Oh, I forgot. Amanda's coming home for the weekend, she called last night. Sorry, I didn't write a note." Then he returns to his cereal as if to hide his embarrassment over the forgotten message.

Bairstow can sense Miriam tighten, and their eyes meet across the room. They've both thought incessantly about Amanda since the shoplifting, searching their minds and hearts about what happened. But there's a part of Bairstow's brain which doesn't want to think about it again. Of course he wants to see her, yet it will revive the ache (will it be there always? he wonders). He can barely remember what it was like with Amanda before--had there been a strain then? No, he can't remember any; their relationship had seemed like any other father-daughter bonding. He is away too much, he understands that. Had he loved his profession too much and neglected his children? He can't answer. He's spent all his spare time with his family, but has it been enough? Yes, he thinks so. Amanda had been a child until recently, and suddenly the change has occured, the rapid metamorphosis to butterfly. It was even difficult to notice the mutation, to note precisely when it occured. Had she emerged from the chrysalis to find something missing, or was it something they'd done to her or that she'd contracted in the process which caused her to suffer this minor flaw? For, Bairstow thinks, it's only shoplifting, it's not a crime against the soul. And

Amanda has good stuff, she'll find the way for herself. He knows it, he feels confident in it. We're not saints, Miriam and I, he thinks, and perhaps Amanda was merely in the wrong place at the wrong time. But he doesn't know, there's still a nagging shadow of doubt.

"It'll be good to see her," says Miriam, placing a soft-boiled egg at Bairstow's place: he hasn't asked for it, but she knows that it's his weakness despite the cholesterol, and he hasn't had one in a long while. "She hasn't been home in six weeks." In her voice Bairstow hears the unspoken words: I love her, I miss her, I worry about her, I can't wait to see her.

Bairstow sits at the table, reading as he eats while Miriam, outside the room, gathers some things together for the boys. He feels a shock reading about the world's violence, which only compounds the gloom he already senses this morning; he'd worried only about June when he awoke this morning, and now other things have crept in...Amanda, difficulties on the surgical service to name two, until the day suddenly seems fraught with challenges. Nevertheless he takes another half cup of coffee from the brewer and finishes the egg. It's a rare morning when he has no surgery, and he intends to savor it. Yet sometimes he feels surgery to be less complicated and more direct and decipherable than the ebb and flow of life in the family: at least he can see what, in his profession, he's dealing with in largely measurable quantities, give or take a few cubic centimeters or milliliters. In the family an outside force can arrive from such a distance as to make the trajectory virtually untraceable--a sudden visit, event, or accident perhaps...or shoplfting. But if science is more stable, it isn't as interesting, either, and too impersonal for his tastes on an exclusive basis. But now and then, he admits it to himself, he feels less suited at home, as if a different language is spoken here, particularly where Amanda is concerned, and he's only glad that Miriam can decipher it.

"You enjoyed your egg?" Miriam asks, returning. Obviously, if he ate it, he enjoyed it, but he knows that she wants something positive from him, and she deserves it. "Thanks, it hit the spot. Will you be home tonight?"

"Of course, Ben. I'm usually home. I like to be home."

That's a fact, she likes her evenings with the family. "And Amanda will be here, too," he responds, looking up from his paper. "I'll try to make sure I get some time free."

"That would be nice. A real family gathering."

They hear the door slam as the twins head out to the bus. Bairstow looks at his watch. "I've got to run, too. Have a good day, Miriam."

"You, too, Ben."

Many of the physicians' wives are gone all the time, Bairstow thinks, to hear the men tell of it. Miriam likes to be home when she isn't out at meetings of one kind or another, but Bairstow thinks she might like it to be gone more, though she seems content cooking, reading and occasionally entertaining women friends. He kisses her, then walks through the downstairs recreation room to the garage, pushes the door opener and starts the Lexus. The solid thrust of the engine restores a certain comfortable hum to his own body, as if the two are hooked to a similar source, and when one starts the other surges as well. Bairstow knows that the luxury vehicle is a vast extravagance in his life for which he feels a little guilty, but not this morning when it's providing the lift, both psychological and actual, that he needs.

He edges into the mounting traffic and realizes that, by delaying, he's missed the chance to beat it. Yet after the meeting he will still have time for rounds, then a decent interval to read completed laboratory tests before the start of morning office hours. June's will not be ready yet. His practice is under control for the moment, the floor supervisor at the other end of his cell phone tells him: Helen Proctor's heart prosthesis is healing nicely. A boy with a tumor, a diabetic with a foot removed, two hernias, a resection of bowel: all doing well. Terry, the boy with Hodgkin's disease, has made an appointment for tests. That's a bonus, at least.

The informal meeting has already begun when Bairstow gets there, and Hanley has been stating his case, his face flushed. Potter is there, and Kulick, and Abernathy, as well as Timkins and Mendino. "I came here," says Hanley, sitting on the edge of the desk in the surgical meeting room which houses the library, "so I could get every other weekend off. And now you tell me..."

"We didn't guarantee it," says Mendino. "At least I didn't."

"I didn't, either," Kulick adds. He is already in his white coat, and Bairstow knows he's an early riser who gets to the hospital at six every morning, sometimes disconcerting the patients and nurses. "I'm on duty often enough as it is, covering..."

"And me, too, among others," says Bairstow, taking a chair at the front of the room, turning it around and straddling it so that he's facing the others. "Can't we all take a day to cover for Hanley? I'll take one, Abernathy the next...all the way down. There's nothing so sacred about my schedule, and I don't mind."

"Well..." begins Timkins. "Is that what all this is about? I suppose..."

"Well..." says Potter. "Except make it during the week because I'm gone on weekends."

"*Every* weekend?" asks Mendino. "What do you do, man? Oh, yes, you ride bicycles. I remember now."

Potter looks him in the eye. "It's about all I do for recreation," he says, not without a hint of malice. "So don't put it down."

Mendino holds up his hands. "Don't misunderstand me..."

Bairstow doesn't have time for this kind of bickering, he wants to see Ebersole. "If it's decided, I've got to leave."

"Well, all right," says Kulick. "Since you all agree..."

It has taken five minutes. They can go on with the rest of this meeting without him, the main point has been resolved. Bairstow has vital things to do down in radiology, that semi-dark world, that twilight domain from which patients love to escape after procedures. He doesn't blame them--he doesn't like it very well, either. He's helped Ebersole with angiograms, even neuro-angiograms where one explores the brain with X-rays after insertion of dye while the patient remains semi-awake. He doesn't like that very well, either. It's eerie, that nether world.

Ebersole is a tall man with straight blond hair which falls to his shoulders, and with gold chains about his neck. Outside the office he wears baggy pants and draws upon a bizarre assortment of T-shirts usually imprinted with ghoulish animals and figures. None of his colleagues can figure them out, which Bairstow thinks might be just as well. He lives in a house, Bairstow has been told, with a giant enlarged picture on the living room wall of an X-ray of his own gallstone, before it was removed. He thinks Ebersole's the least likely medical type he's seen in his entire life, but he practices good medicine. Bairstow has acknowledged to himself on more than one occasion that he'd place himself in Ebersole's hands without question even if he had to stare at those gold chains and have the man's hair fall into his face in the process of having a diagnostic procedure.

Ebersole is drinking coffee in his inner office, gesturing with hands flying as he briefs one of his technicians. Bairstow had to look closely for a minute to allow his eyes to adjust to the gloom down here before he could even find the radiology chief. Everyone dresses in purple, not blue or green as in the operating room and nursing areas, which only serves to make the inhabitants more wraith-like, as if they were in protective coloration like spooks in a cave. Almost as bad as the saffron yellow used in the morgue room, Bairstow thinks with distaste. For some reason he's never entirely trusted Mort Zachary, the morgue supervisor, because he can't imagine what kind of man would spend his life with dead bodies. Bairstow has never examined his own motives for passing *his* hours repairing human bodies, either, but he might have made the immediate distinction, if challenged, that at least *his* bodies are vital and alive, if unconscious...and that makes all the difference.

Ebersole looks up and waves casually to Bairstow. "Hey, man," he says, "how come you aren't in surgery? Oh yeah, I forgot: Thursday, right? Shit, I haven't read the X-rays, forgot it *was* Thursday. You got a minute to look 'em over with me?"

Damn, Bairstow thinks, what was Ebersole up to? Didn't he realize it was Thursday to get his X-ray readings out on time? And didn't he realize that time was valuable in other areas of the hospital where business had to be conducted in a prompt and efficient way? To Bairstow's chagrin, Ebersole finishes his coffee, continuing to chat amiably with the aide as if he, Bairstow, weren't standing right there cooling his heels. Bairstow thrusts his hands into his pocket and moves some change about impatiently to indicate his displeasure, at least giving Ebersole a warning, a small sign, that he's about to erupt like Vesuvius.

But, still talking, Ebersole moves his lanky frame, deposits the cup on the edge of his cluttered desk (Is that the remains of a sandwich? Bairstow wonders, spotting something dried, curled and mummified in a wrapper beside the coffee). Bairstow puts himself determinedly on Ebersole's tail when the man without a word has the audacity to leave the room for the adjoining chamber, a lighter area--or perhaps Bairstow's eyes have at last accommodated themselves to the macabre lighting of this place. Ebersole flips on a switch, and the wall lights up. On a desk before the wall have been placed a stack of X-ray folders, each originally labeled in someone's scrawl, then later typed and mated to a large brown envelope in which the pictures are housed after they've been viewed. Bairstow begins to relax: this is the inner sanctum at last. Ebersole is finally getting to work.

"You had," Ebersole is counting, "ten films in all taken yesterday? Any special order you want to see 'em?"

Bairstow would like to demand to see June's first, but he motions for Ebersole to start at the top, because they're also his patients, and it strikes him as unseemly to consider June's first even if Potter is his partner. A woman who'd been having trouble swallowing is highlighted on the first plate, her glottal region exposed to the all-seeing eye of the X-ray camera. Revealed on the shadowy film is the image of a growth in the soft tissues of her throat, like a small, dark stone,. "It's there," says Ebersole, "you can see it. Size of a pea. Growing pretty fast--I have the earlier film, too."

"Good," says Bairstow, back to business. He examines the plate and nods. "I remember it. Her throat was clear, not a sign of trouble. Treated her symptomatically at the time."

"Sounds reasonable, Ben. You'll call Tenny for this one?" Tenny, they both know, is the staff ENT man who handles this kind of surgery.

"Of course. Does it appear to be operable?"

Ebersole brings his face closer to the screen and nods. "Stinker, though. I'd hate to have to do it. But I don't, do I?" He pretends to wipe away sweat and goes to the next plate, the woman with stomach cancer.

Confirmed is Bairstow's diagnosis: the disease has invaded the surrounding tissues. He shakes his head and wishes the damned machine wasn't so accurate. Why did the thing have the power to allow no alternative, no choice but to reveal one's mortality so graphically for everyone to see? Bairstow will call the oncologist, who can do remarkable things, but may not be able to prolong this woman's life expectancy to what it might have normally been.

The next plate of a nurse whose chief complaint is a cough reveals nothing, only normal, healthy tissue. "You win a few and lose a few," says Ebersole with a sigh--but Bairstow knows that Ebersole wins most often in his X-rays diagnosed in this place. But Ebersole is already holding up the next, revealing the line of a spine, the rib cage with its bent and protective arches, the beginning of the pelvic bones with the light defining the shadows. The X-ray is obviously June's, he can see her name plainly written along the border. "Jeff Potter's wife," says Ebersole matter-of-factly. "I was here when she came in. A real looker, that one."

Bairstow bridles at Ebersole's comments: in this place there's no call for remarks about a patient's attractiveness. What does Ebersole think he's running down here, a charm school? This is a place of medicine, and only that.

"I glanced briefly at these plates myself," Ebersole is running on. "Potter's wife, all that sort of thing." He is standing close to Bairstow now, speaking confidentially, and the scent of his cologne colors the air blue about the two of them, nudging Bairstow's sensitive sinusitis to life again. The damned stuff must be extract of lilac, Bairstow thinks, taking a step away. He's very allergic to lilac, and curbs a sneeze with difficulty. "Potter must be upset, naturally."

"I don't think he knows about her visit. After all, so far it's merely a pain, shortness of breath." Bairstow leans forward to examine the plate more closely, hoping that he's communicated to Ebersole that this is in confidence, at June's request.

Now Ebersole steps back, too, glancing at Bairstow. Bairstow immediately spots the shadow, very faint, in the anterior thorax near the upper lobe of the right lung. "What do you make of it?" he asks, taking a deep breath. "Prognosis, I mean? Is it operable? How do you evaluate it, Max?"

It's the first time in months that Bairstow has called Ebersole by his given name, and the radiologist looks at him sharply, understanding that there is something different in all this from the surgeon who usually remains detached and cool. Of course the woman's husband is Bairstow's partner, and that would account for it. But there's an urgency to his voice that seems to transcend all that, and Ebersole senses that this one has gotten to Bairstow. He tilts his head to one side as he observes the lighted film before him and extends his index finger along the shadow. "Of course, Ben, it may be nothing at all, you can see how faint it is, nothing well-defined. I'd suggest you send her down again and we'll get a better look. But I'd say it might be sticky going because of proximity to the aorta."

Ebersole is right: it'll be very sticky going.

"And you mean it, you don't want this passed on to Potter?"

"I mean it. She hasn't told him, and she wants it kept in confidence."

"Jesus. But I suppose it makes sense because she didn't know what was wrong, and she wants to tell him herself. You want me to contact the patient?"

"Thanks, I'll tell her. She's coming in this morning."

"Sticky wicket." Of course, Ebersole's thinking, Bairstow's told hundreds of people their test results by now, but this one's making him damned unsettled. Understandable. "You want a cup of coffee, Ben?"

"Thanks, I'm a little behind already. Can we finish the films later?"

"Sure, there are only a few more. I'll be around all day."

Bairstow, feeling a little heavier somehow, as if gravity had somehow increased its weight on him, climbs the stairs, then walks to his office. Lousy day. He'd hoped he could relieve June's mind. But, as he has to acknowledge to himself, he'd realized the outcome already, perhaps from the long experience he's had in seeing patients. Deep in his soul of souls he'd known all along that her symptoms were atypical and he'd sensed how the odds stacked up for those symptoms, but he hadn't wanted to acknowledge them. He hates having that inner sense of things about his patients, but there it is...at once a curse and a salvation. From here on he'll have to try to separate his emotions from his judgment if he can, because if he can't, he'll have to disqualify himself from her case, and he doesn't want to do that, either. More than anything, he wants to help June if he can, but her X-rays have shown him just how tricky and painful that might be.

CHAPTER EIGHT

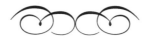

June is already waiting. Val Hobson, interjecting her large frame
through the door, tells him about it. "She's been here fifteen minutes
or so, Dr. Bairstow. In the waiting room."

"Send her in," he tells Val, feeling angry even at Val when he's
merely reacting to the pain of having seen that X-ray. He's well aware
that it'll disrupt her life as well as Potter's, and he's never gotten used
to revealing devastating bad news, especially to friends. "No, wait, I'll
go get her myself."

June, her hair long today, the smooth sweep of it ending just at her
collar, is reading a book, having disdained his waiting room magazines.
She's just turning a page when he spots her, and for a moment she
looks as if she might dash away, a bird poised in flight. No, that's not
correct, he thinks as he looks again, she's merely shifting to get more
comfortable in the chair, ready to continue her reading. He wonders
what book it could be to grasp her attention that way. She's dressed in
a blue suit, well-tailored, with shoulders that seem too padded for her
frame yet make her appear fashionably svelte. She's too thin, Bairstow's

thinking, as he has before, and with those shoulders she's not trying to be chic at all, merely striving to add the illusion of weight to her frame. He's seen that before, too: people losing weight who try to compensate in their clothing.

He walks over to her, and she looks up, her chin tilted toward his face. "Good morning," she says. "It's good of you to see me this morning. Don't you have surgery or something?"

Potter doesn't operate with Bairstow every morning, others fill in on occasion, so she wouldn't know. "I see patients today," Bairstow says. "Let's go to the coffee shop; would you like to? My next patient won't be in for a half-hour at least."

June looks up at him, surprised, then smiles and rises. "It's that bad, is it? You have to buy me coffee to break the bad news?"

Bairstow doesn't answer, there's nothing to say; he merely opens the door and explains to Val that he'll return later. Then they set off down the corridor, where people are changing shift, coming and going. The coffee shop, on the first floor, is barely open, and a volunteer is still arranging things for the day but at least they have boiling water for tea and coffee, and rolls. Bairstow picks up two coffees and two of the rolls, balancing them on a small tray. June has sat herself at a round table in a corner, on one of the ice-cream parlor chairs. Rarely has Bairstow come in here because it seems like such a prissy place, with pink decor...but today it seems like the proper place to come, so unlike the rest of the hospital, so infinitely more cheerful.

Yet Bairstow can't begin immediately. "Traffic heavy?" he asks June. "I'm afraid you came during the rush hour."

She shrugs. "It's not that far, really. I have time, it's not as if I didn't." She takes a sip of the coffee and seems to relax with its warmth. "So what did you see on my X-ray, Ben? You've had a chance to read it?"

He nods. "Yes, just now."

"Well?"

It's the moment he's dreaded, the time when he shatters her life with a few short words, seemingly so moderated, reasonable, measured.

It's true, what Ebersole had implied by his inflection, that he, Bairstow has broken bad news before, but this time he can't make himself feel professional. He can't seem to lower the protective curtain. "There seems to be something there, June. A mere shadow, perhaps nothing to be alarmed about. Ebersole wants you to come in for more pictures."

Bairstow waits for his words to land, to sink in, to settle into June's brain. He feels as if someone has just told *him* that something is lurking inside his own body. He tries to feel as June must feel, but he knows it's impossible: only the victim with the sentence can know what it's like.

June remains calm, barely flinching. Her hands spread casually on the blue wool skirt on her lap, but her fingers seem to stiffen. "Of course," she says. "Of course, Ben."

"I'll go down with you," says Bairstow. "I've just been talking to Ebersole. I'm sure he'll schedule you in today if I make the request."

"That's not necessary. I can wait like everyone else."

"But you're not everyone else. You're my partner's wife. Besides, you're a...friend." Of all the things he wishes to call her, "friend" seems safest.

She contemplates his face. "You're very kind, Ben. You're a kind man."

He's never thought of himself as particularly kind before, he's merely thought that he did as best he could. He knows he's not a bad person, but he's given himself few accolades. Yet it touches him that June envisions him that way. "I wish I'd done something to deserve your praise, June. Would you like to go down after we finish here?" His next patient will be arriving soon.

"You've got time, Ben?"

"A few minutes, anyway. Don't worry, I'll leave when I have to. But you'll come to my office when you've finished?"

"I'd like to." She looks at him, her eyes on his. "You think this... may be serious, don't you?"

He takes a deep breath. "I don't know what to think at this minute. Machines lie, June, they show shadows sometimes which don't exist. I don't want to worry you needlessly, but I think we should...pursue it."

She nods slowly and smiles. "I understand, my friend. But I won't worry if you won't..until there's something to worry about. Is that a bargain?"

Now she's comforting him, a most unlikely position for a doctor. He smiles back. "It's a bargain. But I'm here if you need me.."

"I'm thankful for that."

Bairstow leads her back down to the radiology department. This time they take the elevator because Bairstow doesn't want to tire her; the shock of hearing that one might be harboring a foreign and hostile area of protoplasm must be enough to fatigue and depress anyone. Yet rarely, Bairstow realizes, has he monitored a patient this way, second-guessing her so closely: usually he offers all the suggestions he can and lets it go at that. If a patient doesn't take his advice, it really isn't his fault; if she does, then he tries his level best to provide what cure is in his ability to impart. But he doesn't...can't...allow himself to worry like this.

Ebersole is in the darkroom, the red warning light showing above the door. The room has a cylindrical entryway designed to keep light from entering the inner chamber. They wait for him to emerge, standing together before a bulletin board laden with lists: names of those on call, safety procedures, hospital rules all numbered neatly. Beside them are irreverent cartoons clipped from medical journals.

June turns to Bairstow. "You're nice to take time like this, Ben," she says, moving her head back to see his face. "Yet you didn't believe me when I said you were a nice man. Didn't anyone ever tell you that before?"

Bairstow shrugs. "It just hasn't...seemed...important. I do my job. My feelings--about myself, I mean--don't enter in. They haven't seemed significant."

"Significant? Yes, I see what you mean. Skill at your job has the highest priority. It should, too. Forgive me, that's not what I meant. I wondered how you evaluated yourself, say, on a scale of one to ten."

"I've never evaluated myself that way, on any scale. But, since you ask, I'd put my skill at about eight. Yes, I think so."

"And your integrity?"

"I don't know. I'm an honest person, I'd judge. At least I hope so. As honest as another, I'd say, and perhaps more honest than most."

"I believe you. I trust you. I felt your honesty that night at our house, even though it's hard to say how one senses that about another person. You're compassionate, too. With me, at least."

Bairstow turns to look at her, a hand in his pocket. He feels compassionate, it's true, because he senses her vulnerability. He has the odd feeling that she doesn't feel the full thrust of her situation as much as he does...the devilish weakness of the tissues, so devastating, so capricious. He remembers his conversation with his nurse. "I wouldn't have become a doctor, June, if I hadn't thought I could help a little. Years ago--not very far distant, either--people died young and physicians had pathetically few tools to help. Now we're gaining all the time, although slowly, not half fast enough for..."

At that moment Ebersole emerges from his sanctum, a new set of developed films in his hand. He blinks in the brighter light, then nods at Bairstow.

"Mrs. Potter has agreed to the X-rays you recommend, Max. Can you fit her in this morning?"

Ebersole turns to nod at June. "If you don't mind waiting a few minutes, Mrs. Potter. I have to complete a procedure."

"Of course," answers June. "I don't mind at all. Besides, I have a book with me." She holds it up briefly, and Bairstow can see that it's a book on clinical psychology.

"Then have a seat," says Ebersole. He indicates a group of chairs against the wall. "I won't be long." He turns and strolls up the hall, ambling at his usual lackadaisical pace.

"I can wait with you," says Bairstow. "At least for five minutes or so." His first patient, old Mrs. Marlow, is invariably late, and has kept him waiting each of the four times he's seen her in the last month.

"No." June is shaking her head. "I wouldn't think of it, Ben. You've spent too much time with me already."

"I haven't, but it's true, I do have to leave. I'll see you when you're finished." To his astonishment, his own words carry in his ear the sound of anticipation at seeing her soon, and a reluctance at relinquishing her here. "I'm afraid that the X-rays won't be ready for a while.. But...why don't you join me for lunch? This is an easier day for me."

He can see June looking at him, her eyes opened wider now, and he doesn't know what she will say. Perhaps she'll think he has no right to do this, to be asking for her company in such an open way, that it's somehow improper. But who gives a damn, anyway? He can see her making the decision, her eyes flickering slightly.

"Why, I'd love to, Ben. I could meet you in your waiting room when I've finished if you'd like."

Whatever he'd wanted to say to her, he decides, can wait. They will have leisure time together later. And whatever is on those X-rays won't plague them quite yet because there is nothing definite, and for a short while longer they can turn their backs on the possibilities. He admires her for that, the ability to hold those possibiities in obeyance: it's a quality he's observed in many of his patients, that coolness under stress, at once astonishing and commendable. June will, of course, tell Potter tonight and he will stand by her and give her support, but in the interim he'll keep himself available. Or at least he rationalizes so, but something is telling him that her company has become so pleasant that it has become an end in itself. And if she had objected she could have refused his invitation for lunch, after all.

He leaves her sitting in one of the stiff chairs in Ebersole's waiting room, trying to read in the dim light of a small lamp beside the chair. She waves to him briefly, then returns her attention to the book, frowning as she tries to pick out the words. Bairstow springs up the stairs, almost bowling over a young aide carrying bloods to pathology, also located in this nether region of the hospital. He suddenly feels unaccountably content, inexplicably full of well-being. Yet his waiting room is already filling: Mrs. Marlow, who he's evaluating for phlebitis, on whom he's operated twice in the past, gives him a disapproving eye and pointedly looks at her watch despite the fact that this is the first time he's known her to be on time. Yet she has a right to be miffed, Bairstow thinks, but right now he can't even find the necessary conscience inside himself to feel guilty. What a sorry state he's come to. Two other patients sit talking together on the other side of the room; they look up briefly as he walks across the carpeted floor. Jan Valenti, gossiping with Val, quickly adjusts her uniform. The office has been poised, waiting for him, and now the morning will begin.

The steady trek of patients across his floor commences: an electrician with complications from ulcer surgery, a tiny baby with a strangulated hernia, a man requiring a skin graft, a woman with a shadow in the breast on X-ray. One after the other they progress across his tweed carpet, which the salesman had told him so many years ago "would virtually last forever" but is now showing incipient wear and tear.

Bairstow feels that he, too, has been showing a little of the same wear and tear, but lately his condition has lifted somewhat: he's been aware of a rejuvenation, a renewal in energy. Where it comes from he hasn't a clue. Yet, he should cheer his patients, he thinks, so whatever causes the upturn in his voice is welcome. It was the same tone which had surprised Val Hobson recently, when he'd seen her looking at him curiously. Time for everyone to realize that there's life at forty, that his life is at the prime, not dribbling down the other side of the hill. Yet all the time he's aware of June, sitting down in X-ray, tensely awaiting another look-see from Ebersole's machine. He wonders what she's thinking--does she speculate on what he's doing now, as he does with her? But she doesn't even know what he does: to begin to imagine his steps back and forth between his office and the hospital, for his life is full of such backward and forward, repetitive motion. His life is more involved here than is Potter's. A tracing of his movements would defy even her speculation, but perhaps she does speculate, nonetheless. Perhaps she pictures his face, as he does hers, unbidden; even now he can see the waves of hair falling over her cheeks and down onto her shoulders. Does she think of him in his office, dressed in his white coat, or in surgery, covered so impersonally in formless green robes? Perhaps. But maybe she doesn't think of him at all. She is too involved in her own world to spare thoughts of him, and he is silly to waste time like this wondering how she conducts her reveries when she is away from him. Why, he doesn't know half the time what Miriam thinks about in her days away from him, either, though she relates what deeds were accomplished in her meetings and home hours. Sometimes, he regrets that he's fatigued and listens with half an ear. What had Miriam said this morning, that she and her organization were trying to save an old landmark, the Cogden House, from being razed to make way for a parking lot? Bairstow hadn't been entirely sure what the Cogden House looked like. Yet now he's putting himself into the role of clairvoyant, trying to imagine what June might be thinking about him, how he appears to her in her mind's eye! He pulls himself up short: he has work to do.

Mrs. Marlow has no complications from surgery so he dismisses her with a prescription: he'll not need to see her for another year. The electrician has just moved back to this area after a period away, during which time his wife died from a stroke. Now he wants to reunite with old friends and relatives. While he was away, a local surgeon repaired his ulcer, but had sutured his intestine at the same time. He'd almost starved by the time he came back to Bairstow for help. Bairstow himself had required the man to go through a battery of tests before he'd been able to pinpoint the problem and go after it. Now the man is finally recovered; Bairstow prods his abdomen a last time, then helps him off the table. When the electrician is dressed, they shake hands... it will probably be the last time they will meet. The electrician hasn't requested Bairstow to testify in court against the other physician who stapled part of his intestine, so he apparently isn't planning to sue, even though the other physician's actions were negligent. But Bairstow, to tell the truth, is relieved because he dislikes testifying in court--to be sure, he's done it often enough, but he hates damning other doctors, and he always feels pretty dejected afterward. He's begun to dislike the peremptory challenging of physicians for every imputed misjudgment, every picayune slip an eager and avaricious lawyer can possibly dredge up. Most doctors are not scavengers nor opportunists in Bairstow's view, but merely human. Sure, he's run across a bastard or two, but he thinks the entire profession is taking it on the chin, that it's being maligned far beyond its transgressions. When, he wonders, will the lawyers step forward and be charged for every error they've committed and for the endless grief they've caused so many in his profession?

By now, Bairstow thinks as he watches the electrician leave, June should have been ushered into Ebersole's X-ray room, there to be undressed and photographed again. This time Ebersole will position her in a variety of contorted poses to get at that lung area where they'd seen the shadow. He sympathizes for the distress all this will cause her, for the indignity of it. This time they may find nothing, nothing at all, when the machine levels its energy at the specific area beneath her rib. He hopes to God that's the way it will be, that his dire thoughts will prove unfounded.

So Bairstow frets in his office, trying to apply himself to immediate problems. The tiny baby before him, held by its mother, glares over at him furiously and breaks into cries. The mother, a Peruvian Indian who stands bolt upright beside his desk, moves aside her voluminous, embroidered robes to expose her breast for the child to feed. Bairstow's used to the woman nursing her child here in his office by now, for she's done it on every visit. It's rather nice, he thinks, that the woman is so unself-conscious with him; her gap-toothed concentration is almost endearing. She speaks English well enough to be understood when her words are coupled with sign language, nods, or vigorous shakes of the head. The woman wears a long, fat pigtail queuing down her back, tied with a ribbon. Her robes appear handmade with a geometric pattern and a bright blue stylized bird interwoven on the purple cloth. The woman, as she has before, glances about herself quickly, running her eye over Bairstow's furniture--the mahogany desk and pile rug and cushioned chairs. Bairstow knows that she disapproves, he can see it in the stiff way she holds her head and back. It's far too fancy for her tastes. But he can't help it, she can disapprove all she wants because he furnishes it as it is for the convenience of his patients so it doesn't look like Ebersole's cell.

Bairstow motions for her to sit down again, but she shakes her head instead and hands the baby to Bairstow, sweeping it from her breast. The baby begins to scream again at the removal of its solace, and Bairstow suddenly finds himself in total possession of a plump, drooling, pear-shaped, black-haired, olive-skinned infant, wriggling like a little pig to escape him.

For a minute Bairstow thinks he's going to drop the little child, and clutches so hard to insure its safety that the baby screeches all the louder. The woman at last sits down, having abdicated her responsibility to Bairstow on the assumption that the white doctor knows what he's doing. Bairstow knows that nothing could be farther from the truth, and without a word lays the infant on his desk amid the charts and reports and correspondence while he figures what to do next. He'd intended for the mother to take the child to his examining room before she'd suddenly appeared at the door, but now the die is cast and his desk has been miraculously transformed into an examining table. He realizes that his face must betray his astonishment when he looks at the woman and finds her grinning at him. The smile is so ingenuous that he can't help but smile back, mostly at himself for the pickle he's gotten into, but he dutifully unwraps the baby until he's down to the tiny scar he himself placed there a month ago when he operated on the child for strangulated hernia.

He feels about the tiny incision, which is pink and healthy, with the baby screeching at him all the while. The mother has taken to rocking back and forth in her chair, carefree now while another watches her offspring, and one as capable as this white doctor. Bairstow finishes, rewrapping the baby as if it were a present or a dinner napkin, and hands it back to its mother. At last he's recovered his bearings. "Your baby's fine, just fine," he tells the rocking mother. "All's well. Can you understand?"

The woman rises and nods back. She tucks the baby onto a hip and walks out the door in her flat-footed gait, rolling her hips outward as she goes, then turns back and smiles. In response, Bairstow waves--it's the only salute he can think of that she'll readily understand. He will probably never see her again, either, since she's here fleetingly on a peace mission of some kind.

He greets another man in the hall outside his office and leads him into the examining room. Bairstow has had the man as a patient for years, has recently done some skin grafting on an area of his leg that wouldn't heal. The man, Mr. Grumman, is old and feeble and, Jan says, has taken to walking outside the nursing home. Apparently he's clever as a fox at escaping. His son is with him, Jan informs Bairstow, but already Mr. Grumman has given him the slip when he went to the men's room. Today for some reason, it touches Bairstow that this man is wandering loose about the place trying to find a door ajar to let him out of his cage. Life can be a cage sometimes, Bairstow thinks, and Mr. Grumman isn't the first of his patients to try to find a way out. Bairstow hopes he never gets to this pass, where life is almost intolerable and he wants to escape its constraints.

Eventually Grumman is located by his son wandering the hall outside the men's room, is examined, leaves, and the next patient and the next have come and gone. It is late in the morning, and his hours have been unusually long today because of walk-ins. He's consumed with concern that June has gone, that she's been bored waiting for him, that the entire episode has been a mirage. Perhaps he really hadn't seen her earlier and she hadn't consented to have lunch with him at all, it's merely a figment of his overworked brain. He rushes once again into the waiting room, his white coat flapping--and there she is after all, engrossed in the same book she'd been reading earlier. He alters the hurried pace of his step as he approaches her, takes a breath and grasps her arm gently. "I'll be only a minute," he says, trying to hide his consternation. "Be right back. Don't go away."

She looks up at him and smiles. "I'm in no hurry, Ben. Please don't rush. And I wouldn't think of going away."

He relaxes, shedding some of his anxiety while he removes his white coat, hangs it in the closet, and heads to Ebersole's domain to discover what June's X-ray reveals.

CHAPTER NINE

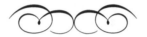

The hospital environs are bereft of restaurants, and Bairstow has had something special in mind. He tells Val Hobson to call his first two afternoon patients and ask them to delay; then he takes June by the arm and steers her toward his car, opening the door for her and seeing that she's settled inside. He's reminded with a pang that he rarely opens the door for Miriam these days, and vows to do better by her from now on.

June seems preoccupied. "It went all right?" he asks, turning toward her as he starts the engine. "What did Ebersole say?" Ebersole had been in his darkroom developing the morning films when Bairstow arrived at the radiologist's office earlier, but maybe he'd given a preliminary hint to June about what her plate had revealed. She presses against the soft fabric of the seat and turns toward him so that he can see the contour of her forehead and the smooth skin of her cheek. "He didn't say anything. He flapped his beads at me and took the pictures. He rolled me around the table and got laterals and dorsals and all kinds of shots from above and sideways. Now I know what a model must go through with all those odd poses."

Bairstow had known it would be unpleasant, but he hadn't reckoned with Ebersole's almost monomaniacal thoroughness: it made him a good doctor, of course, but was enough to drive a normal person batty.

"You're worried," June says, continuing to look at him. "You think I can't handle it if the X-rays show something more."

"You aren't expected to handle everything. How can you, June? We're all human, after all, and we've got our melting points." Bairstow hasn't said it in quite this way to other patients, the ones he's treating for debilitating illnesses, and he makes the mental note that he will from now on. Too often he's left most of the major issues for patients and their relatives to cope with, and now he understands how wrong that is. He should shoulder more of the emotional baggage of their illnesses and vows to do so in the future.

"But I *can* handle myself, Ben. Did you know that I was married... before Jeff, I mean?"

Bairstow takes his eyes from the road to look at her. He shakes his head. "I had no idea. Potter never told me."

"Jeff is pretty self-contained. I mean, I know he'd never let on, even with you."

"You were divorced?" Somehow Bairstow is surprised again that Potter had never let a word drop inadvertently at one time or another--but then, Bairstow has only recently met June and entered the private domain of Potter's family

June shakes her head, a quick, tense gesture as if trying to make the memory pass. "They were killed, my husband and my son. In a car accident, just like that. Here one moment and gone...the next." Despite her earlier bravado, her voice modulates and then almost breaks. "I'm sorry," she gasps, "I thought I was over all that. It was four years ago. I thought I could manage anything after that and here I go letting loose again."

He stares at the road ahead, feeling her pain. "I'm sorry, June. I didn't know about the marriage or the child. I only knew you don't have children now."

"Thanks, Ben. Jeff wishes we had kids, he talks about it all the time. We've tried since we've been married, but to no avail." She reaches for a kleenex in her handbag, a small pouch which she's placed on the floor beside her feet. "I think Jeff blames me somehow, even though I'd gotten pregnant by my first husband...and Jeff's not sterile; we've had all the tests. But I ovulate oddly, and for a while after the accident I got too thin, almost like an anorectic, and I understand that anorectics are often barren, at least until they gain weight."

Bairstow rides along, listening to the sound of June's voice; even if the words are full of sorrow for her, they soothe him just because she is beside him.

"Well, I regained most of the weight, and I still can't get pregnant. One day soon we'll have to go in for more tests, I suppose, but we keep putting it off. Every month I think that something will happen, but it never does."

Children can be very difficult to raise; it isn't a bed of roses, Bairstow is thinking, his mind picking Amanda from the list of situations he must deal with this week. Then he feels a pang, knowing how much he loves her and remembering the good times he's had with his children over the years. He can also imagine the ache for one without offspring, which would be much worse. Yet raising children takes energy and patience, and sometimes he's felt as if he should have had more of both and didn't when the vital moments came in his relationship with his own offspring.

"You look very serious," says June with a smile, observing his face as he negotiates the car down a side road. "I'm afraid I jogged a sore memory. Did I say something?"

Bairstow shakes his head. "I was thinking of my daughter when you spoke of not having children. When she got into trouble for shoplifting, it was agony getting things settled. I thought Miriam would die. But our kids are really all right, all of them."

June nods. "I *know* they're a challenge, you don't have to tell me. My mother says I was a handful, growing up. I don't remember that, of course, because I was convinced I was an angel." She follows the remark with a laugh, and Bairstow, the tension broken, laughs with her. He has an impulse to hug her, to pull her close to him, but luckily he's got his hands on the wheel and the moment passes, though he can still feel the warmth and promise of the impulse.

Bairstow leaves the car for the attendant to park; it's the only restaurant in the city with a valet service, and although Bairstow comes here rarely, he is always a little awed despite himself. It makes him feel successful, as if at last the poor parochial boy has come into his own.

"You're trying to impress me," says June as Bairstow takes her arm and leads her through the carved wooden doors, standing open before them and revealing the elegant foyer. The maitre d' is already on his way over, smiling solicitously and obviously ready to please. Bairstow feels that he's not known here and they'll probably sit him at some inconvenient table against an inner wall, so he's astonished to find that they're being led forward toward a bank of long windows facing out onto a long, sloping, verdant lawn.

"Well," says June, "I *am* impressed, you can stop now. What a lovely view! Did you ever see a lawn so green?"

Bairstow can feel his own pleasure, observing June so delighted. "You'll have to ask Potter to bring you here sometime. It's not as expensive as it looks, really. And it *is* a treat, you feel a little like a king; 'Monarch of all I survey.' Isn't there a poem that goes something like that?"

June laughs, a charmed, childlike sound. "You're reciting poetry to me, Ben? I never would have thought it. Why, I can't remember when anyone's quoted poetry to me before. Not for a very long time, anyway."

Bairstow, in spite of himself, finds his face flushing. "I'm far from a poet, June. Sometimes I think I'm pretty near illiterate in anything beside medicine. There never seems any time for...no, that's a terrible excuse, I'm ashamed to say it. Miriam thinks I'm a disaster when it comes to culture, and she's absolutely right."

The waiter arrives, an impeccably dressed man wearing a red fitted jacket with gold braid trim. They order drinks. "I hope," says June, "that you don't treat all your patients like this. You'd have the biggest practice in the city by far, but I suspect you'd go broke rather rapidly. Incidentally, I'm no good at culture, either. I try to paint--you already know that--but I'm nowhere near good enough."

"For what? Your work appears extraordinary to me. I already know that much."

Bairstow contemplates her while she's sipping her drink: she holds the long-stemmed glass delicately in her long fingers, bending her head to the glass. June seems perfectly suited to this place, but she's not as sophisticated as many of the other women he can observe in this room, wearing hats and low-cut blouses and sitting archly talking to companions. June seems almost as if she's on an outing, a child unused to picnics, ingenuous about her enjoyment. That enthusiasm, evident in all her motions, transfers itself to Bairstow. At least, he thinks, she's been momentarily diverted from the ordeal she's been experiencing since the machine delineated that faint tracing on her lung. Bairstow had intended as much, the reason for this foray having been founded partly on that hopeful goal. Yet, Bairstow thinks, he's the one who needed the cheering-up since she is obviously handling it in stride. Perhaps she has become a survivor after the ordeal of her husband and baby dying so tragically. And maybe she has of necessity contracted a little of the fatalism a doctor must learn if he is to survive. But he knows that Potter will be devastated when he returns and that this foray is the least he can do.

He finds her looking at him. "A penny for your thoughts," she says. "But I may not want to know. You don't like to let on what's going through your head, do you?"

Bairstow nods. "You're right, I don't."

"Why not? Do you mind if I ask?"

"Of course not. It's just that I've never trusted another's opinion. I have to make up my own mind in surgery, and in others things as well. It's been that way since I was a child. If I make a mistake, I want it to be mine alone."

"Do you think Dr. Ebersole made a mistake about the shadow on my plate, Ben?"

"About the shadow...no. About what it signifies..."

"You'd give me your honest opinion?"

He feels her pressing him, and he has to resist his own impulses to give her hope when he knows very well she may have a real problem. "Yes, I would. I'd never keep anything from a patient...unless she didn't want to know."

"But you know that I do...want to know, I mean."

He reaches his hand forward, and is about to grasp hers but again resists the impulse. "I'm sorry, June, I'm not being merely evasive. I never speculate, either. I deal in realities, not possibilities. Conjectures make for bad medicine. Tests will answer your question but I can't."

"That's what Jeff says. Forgive me for prying, I didn't want you to speculate. I know it's an unwritten rule and that I broke it. I don't mean to sound frantic, either, because I'm really not, although I'm... concerned, naturally."

He finds himself touched by her again, and for a moment glances down at his lunch, the chicken divan and fresh peas and rolls which he's been barely able to touch; they stand neglected as are June's asparagus and toast points. Neither of them is hungry, the curse of it in this epicurean palace, but it almost seems unimportant. "I admire your reserve and obvious strength, June," he says. "Some of my patients would be frantic, contemplating problems of their own health. Sometimes I feel that my mouth is sealed at all the wrong times...maybe from disuse in talking about my own feelings but probably from a real sense of inadequacy to help. But I really wanted to help in some way, and so..."

"You took me to a lovely lunch, Ben. What could be nicer?"

It's true, here they are together, he's escorted his partner's wife to lunch. He wonders idly if Miriam's been taken to lunch by a man.

Perhaps she has. Once, a few years ago, he might have wanted to duel the fellow over it, but now it has little significance in the scheme of things when the pattern of his life is established. Over coffee, Bairstow leans his elbows on the table and looks over at June. She appears relaxed, lunch has gone well. He savors the inner content he is feeling; yet this afternoon he is on duty and understands from long experience that he'll be confronted with many small emergencies and perhaps one or two large ones. "I'll call," he says. "After I've been in touch with Ebersole. Or would you rather I contacted Potter? He can decipher the findings for you, because for a layman they're apt to be mumbo-jumbo and signify very little."

"Please call me. Jeff's away on a bicycle trip."

"I'd forgotten. You'll be home?"

"Yes. All afternoon. Thanks, Ben, for everything. And I'm sorry... for all the trouble."

"But I never said that, June. You're not causing any trouble."

"I know, but I feel so sometimes. You have so much strength, and I envy that. More than Jeff, I think: he escapes by training for races. You stand your ground and fight. That makes you aware--do you realize that--that you're ready for what comes. You anticipate, but you have to cover up more, too. I don't know which is best, escaping or protecting one's self for the next assault."

Bairstow shakes his head: he's never thought of himself as ready for the blows that come, but he can see what June means. It's true that medicine is a continual assault, that one's senses and sensibilities are constantly under bombardment. He still hasn't reached the stage of constant fatigue that his older colleagues profess to feel, but he knows that after a while one can't grapple, not with the hours, but with the emotional overload. It must be so with teachers, too, or any other profession; except that in medicine, patients die.

They must leave; Bairstow knows that his appointments for his first patients must be coming closer, his inner clock is ticking away. After these years with so many patients coming and going constantly, he's developed an inner sense of urgency, as has anyone who sets their lives in time frames.

June has seen it in his face. "I know we must leave, Ben," she says. "Our few minutes of high happiness are passing."

The expression makes Bairstow smile: "High happiness" is perhaps just right, time spent elevated in spirit and in haute cuisine at the same time.

"I mean it," June continues, seeing his smile. "It's been one of the high spots of my week...no, my year. Maybe even my life, who knows?"

When Bairstow looks at June, he knows that she means it. It's the same for him, this short time. Some moments, he thinks, have their own significance, and one doesn't have to explain them. Like moments in surgery, some are spent with intense involvement, and those can occur even when things are going well, when there's no alarm, when there's a heightened awareness of the intrinsic coalescing of vital, even random or unconscious forces. Today has been like that.

Just inside the magnificent stone foyer, within view of the mammoth carved doors, they wait for the car; Bairstow has handed his ticket to the young man in the not-too-well-fitting uniform who rushes about finding the parked automobiles and brings them to the front portico. They wait patiently inside the door. Bairstow has no wish to hurry this moment, nor apparently does June. She stands beside him, her shoulders held slightly forward inside the beige all-weather coat she had been carrying when she'd arrived. Now it has turned cooler and the air is misting slightly. They can see the roadway turning wet outside the tall windows. June is close to him, her arm almost touching his coat. He can smell her perfume and see the highlights of her hair. Cars come and go outside: apparently the restaurant is short of help today, which explains the attendant's rushing about--some customers are parking their own cars, swinging through the doors as Bairstow and June wait, so close together. She moves her hands to her pockets, her elbows now resting against Bairstow's arm. Rain drips lightly from the roof beyond the entryway onto the roadway on the far side of the portico.

Just then Bairstow catches a familiar sight, a quick flash of movement which somehow registers on a receptive part of his brain. He doesn't have to move his head: she is in the direct line of his gaze. He takes a deep breath as the young woman steps from the car not ten paces from him. "What...?" says June, sensing a change in Bairstow's mood. "Who is that?"

Bairstow turns toward the woman, now just outside the oaken doors, a man having joined her. "Amanda!" he exclaims. "What in God's earth are you doing here?"

The young woman stops in her tracks, her mouth fallen open. She flushes. June looks at Bairstow and realizes instantly who the woman is: she has precisely the same coloring as her father and the same shocked expression in the deep brown eyes and tilt to the angle of the chin.

Yet she seems not quite so ill at ease as Bairstow. "Why...hello, father. I guess I can ask the same question. What on earth are *you* doing here?"

The two stare at each other a moment longer, the man accompanying Amanda seeming momentarily off balance.

Bairstow recovers himself with difficulty, and for a moment is almost unable to talk. "June, this is my daughter, Amanda. Believe it or not."

June inclines her head and smiles, but Amanda makes no effort to introduce her companion, a dark-complected man appearing years her senior. Instead she turns to him haughtily. "Don't you think we'd better go now, Mario?" She makes a gesture as if to pull him along, impatiently plucking at his sleeve.

"Not so quick, young lady," says Bairstow. "I thought you were coming home tomorrow. What are you doing here today? And that dress"--he indicates her plum-colored wool arranged to display Amanda's ample bosom--"doesn't that belong to your mother?"

By now Amanda has her fingers grasping her companion's coat. "Mario, if you don't come this minute, I'm going in by myself." She is already through the entryway and heading for the main room of the restaurant. "Mario!"

"Excuse," says Mario, and in a twinkling has shoved past them, just behind Amanda.

Bairstow stands looking after them, a stricken look on his face, feeling utterly assaulted, as if the very air has turned dark. "What the hell do you suppose she's doing here? And dressed like that? Why, I should go in there and drag her home. What does she think she's doing, anyway?" He feels strangely impotent in this public place, frustrated and embattled.

June slips her arm through his. "It's all right, Ben. It's all *right.* You *can't* drag her home, she's almost an adult." She pulls him gently toward the door. "Do you want to walk around for a while?"

He doesn't respond but, frustrated, allows June to tug him out the door, as if giving direction to a rudderless ship. "Do you want me to drive?" she asks. "I'll be glad to, you know."

"Did you see the dress she was wearing?" Bairstow persists. "It's her mother's, she just bought it. Why, she must have sneaked home...and that necklace--do you know that I paid a fortune for it ten years ago? Our anniversary. Now she's taken it, *stolen* it, no doubt."

"Give me the keys," June says, reaching for the leather case in Bairstow's hand. "My first husband had a Lexus. I'm used to one."

Obediently, he hands them over. "Wait until Miriam finds out. My God, she'll have a stroke."

The attendant is staring at them, but Bairstow follows June's directive, settles into the car, then pulls his door shut. She steps her foot on the accelerator, and they take off down the circular drive.

"What the hell do you suppose she was doing here?" Bairstow goes on. "And who was that creepy guy? I know damn well she's up to no good."

June is moving the car rapidly away from the hilly area where the restaurant is located down into the valley, taking right turns, then waiting for a set of lights. "She was probably doing the same thing we were," she says. "Having lunch. And you can find out who he is if you really want to know. But it won't help to make that kind of decision when you're this upset."

"She was released on probation," Bairstow persists. "The judge said she had to report to the court for a year. That man she was with is up to no good."

"But you don't *know* that, Ben. Maybe he's a friend. Maybe he's even...a teacher or someone."

"I'd hate to think what *he'd* teach her."

The trees clear magically before them, and they are entering a park where tall trees soar high above them, and in a minute the car is proceeding beside a small river perhaps fifty feet away in which large stones prompt the water to eddy and swirl into separate cascades. For the first time Bairstow seems to take note of his surroundings. "Where are we, for God's sake? Where have you taken me, June?"

June laughs at him. "Along the river, haven't you ever come here? I come whenever...I feel upset. It attracts migratory birds this time of year--see, there are Canada geese out there now. And rowers."

"But I have patients to see, and..."

"Hospital patients, you said, you can make rounds on them later. Besides, you wouldn't make sense to them in this state. We won't be here long. And we're not far from the hospital, not more than three miles. Sometimes Jeff rides his bike here on the path, or comes at noon, to eat a sandwich I pack for him."

Bairstow is beginning to simmer down. He stuffs his hands into his pockets, and they walk slowly up the path. Geese arise from the water below them, their great wings beating against the air to give them displacement against the air currents. They are so breathtaking that, in watching them, Bairstow finds his anger subsiding. He stands silently on the path, observing the birds on the water and flapping in the air.

"You want to walk a while?" June asks, glancing up at him. He nods and they continue down the path. After a minute he catches her hand and holds it tightly in his. "Thanks," he says. "I behaved like a fool and demented idiot. I'm sorry. I don't know how the hell it happened." Wasn't he supposed to be the detached doctor, calm in his decisions?

They continue to stroll up the pathway, Bairstow taking in deep breaths. He feels as if his brain has been on fire. "It's the waste," he begins again. "Amanda has been given everything we could think of to make her happy. She had every lesson you could imagine: guitar, piano, dance, aerobics. Because *she* wanted them, not because Miriam and I forced her. She complains of our wealth, of my car, saying it's so ostentatious. I think it's one of the most beautifully built machines of this century, and I'm proud of it. I value it; I repaired car engines when I was a kid to get through college. I paid dearly for it, in midnight hours of work, in training, in sweat. What does Amanda value? Not the things, obviously, that we've tried to give her, to make possible for her? What is she doing with her life? Stealing underwear and her mother's jewels?"

June shakes his hand lightly, a small, impatient gesture. "Ben, she's going to school, that's plenty. She's paying her fine. And just because you saw her at that restaurant..."

"I don't like it. I don't like that man."

"Does it make any difference whether you like him or not? It's *her* life. If she chooses to steal underwear and go to jail, that's her life, too. Didn't you say she's eighteen? That's the age of consent, you know."

"Still..."

"I wasn't crazy about the way the man looked, either. But you don't have the right to make derogatory comments, don't you see?"

"While she's living at my house..."

"But she isn't, she's living at prep school..." June smiles at his distraught face. "You're providing an education for her, and that's nice. Lots of people tell their kids to finance it on their own, because they can't afford it. You're offering the option to Amanda." She takes a breath. "I think you're going to have to let her go, Ben. You hold on like bloody death. She's entitled to make a few mistakes on her own. I know I did."

"Not stealing."

"No, not stealing."

Bairstow doesn't answer, and they continue walking. Finally, after minutes of silence, he turns to her. "What makes you so sure of this? How do you know so much? Where did you hear all of this?"

She brushes a wisp of hair from her cheek. "I guess I went through it, too. My father was a strict man. I didn't even know him that well, he was so busy. That's often the way with doctors, I'm used to it. I had a brother who died in the Vietnam War--did I tell you that? After that, my father preferred to bury himself in his profession to being with my mother and me, at least that's the way I interpreted it. But now I think he was simply making a name for himself, it was his ambition. Why shouldn't he? That kind of dedication takes time. I loved him. But perhaps Amanda is merely rebelling and this is her way. She's entitled to her rebellion; maybe it's necessary for her future growth. But whatever she's doing doesn't have anything to do with you and Miriam because she's a big girl now."

Bairstow watches her face. "You're saying that if she should get into trouble again I shouldn't intercede because it's her responsibility...?"

"I'm saying that maybe you should lighten up a bit."

They turn to walk back. Bairstow is staring at the path beneath their feet, his hands in his pockets.

"You're angry?" June asks. "I'm afraid I've meddled where I have no right."

"No, it helps. I was thinking what a relief it is to allow someone independence. I always had it as a child, so maybe I was lucky. Men experience it more than women, I'm sure of it. Maybe I've forgotten to notice that Amanda has grown up. She still makes me furious...every time I think of her back at the restaurant, but I'll try for some kind of perspective. If I can."

Within minutes they're back on their circuit through the park, around the shore of the river and the adjacent little lake, to the car. "You're going to tell your wife we saw Amanda?" June asks.

Bairstow shakes his head.

"Because it will upset her about Amanda?" June asks. "Or because we were at the restaurant together?"

Bairstow has opened the door of the car for her. "Both. I think I'm deeper into this than I thought. I don't want to stop, June. I've enjoyed being with you."

"And I with you, Ben. Thank you. You're a good man, I told you... and a fine doctor. It's an unbeatable combination in my book."

He drives her back to the hospital, to her car, then watches her disappear down the long hospital drive. For a moment he almost feels bereft, the feeling is that intense. But he has a busy day. He turns and walks into the hospital. It's time to find out, whether he wants to or not, what Ebersole found on June's X-ray plate.

CHAPTER TEN

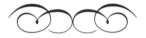

*E*bersole is nowhere to be seen, but his assistant, a short, squat man named Breslin, is sitting at his desk entering diagnostic notes into a computer.

"Is Max around?" Bairstow asks. "I'd like to talk to him."

Breslin jerks his thumb toward the darkroom. "He's in there. Ought to be out soon, though. Hell of a busy morning."

"I'll wait," says Bairstow. He sits down in a stiff metal tubular chair nearby with a worn back and even more threadbare arms. Where does Ebersole dredge up this stuff, he wonders, it's unreclaimable junk. He picks up a magazine whose cover has a picture of a sailboat with a pretty girl in the bow. Bairstow is startled because the woman looks a little like June. Maybe I'm imagining things, he thinks: I'm seeing June everywhere. Is it merely concern for her welfare, or is this getting out of hand? He passes his hand across his forehead, then locks both hands behind his head. He doesn't know the answer to that one but he's got his suspicions. Strange doings, he thinks, for an M.D. in his prime and pretty much set in his ways. He compresses his lower lip. Maybe aging a little, but not aging *that* much, and hopefully not that much set in his ways, either. Midlife crisis? Dear God, what kind of a crisis is that?

Briefly he thinks of Amanda, and finds his anger to have mostly dissipated. He decides he won't worry about her, he'll do as well as he can by her, but she's responsible for her own fate. Perhaps it's true, as June said, that one can do only so much for another. Then it's time to quit and let that other take responsibility.

He's sitting there, hands behind his head staring at the ceiling, when Ebersole emerges from the darkroom dressed in his purple garb. Not noticing Bairstow, Ebersole starts to walk past Breslin on his way to the interior of the department when Breslin stops him and points with his pen toward Bairstow. In a moment Ebersole has furled his long frame into the second chair.

"You're haunting the place," says Ebersole. "You're pretty worried about that case, Bairstow." It's neither a question nor a flat statement.

Bairstow nods. "Potter's wife, yes."

Ebersole looks at him. "I have the feeling that she's more than Potter's wife. But you can stop me if I'm getting out of line."

"Then stop, you're getting out of line."

"All right. But I've had a few flings in my life, too, you know."

"Well, *I* haven't. And it isn't a fling. She's a nice woman having some problems right now--and Potter's not around to help out. Damn his hide! He's into bike racing every spare minute, so she can't talk to him about it just when she needs him."

"Why not? What's she afraid of?"

"Cut it out, Max! She's not afraid of anything. She doesn't want to upset him, that's all, when he's in some kind of race. She's a considerate woman...."

"Yes? You sound like her press agent."

Bairstow stands up. "I came down to look at her films, Ebersole, and I'd like to get on with it, if you don't mind."

Ebersole slowly rises, too, then places his hand on Bairstow's shoulder. "Give the film ten more minutes. Sorry, friend, I'm a genius at running off at the mouth. To make you feel better--half the hospital isn't talking to me. I say the wrong thing at the wrong time. Oh, I enjoy it but for some reason others don't. Tell me what you think about Potter's wife."

Ten minutes? Ebersole's taking his bloody times today but Bairstow's had those days, too. "She's too thin, Max, and too pale. I'd speculate it isn't simply anemia..."

Ebersole scratches his head thoughtfully. "Actually, she struck me the same way, as if something wasn't quite right..."

The attendings back in medical school used to maintain that they could diagnose a case by the way a patient, man or woman, walked down the corridor. Bairstow thought they were self-important braggarts then, but now that he's had almost as many years of experience as they had then, he's wondering if they might not have been right after all.

A timer goes off. "Come along," says Ebersole. "They're ready. You want to see the others, too?"

"As long as I'm here." He's sent two other patients to Ebersole for X-rays.

The films are still warm from the developing process. Ebersole checks the names of the patients and referring physicians against the markers, then places three of the films against the illuminating wall. The first are June's pictures, all right, taken in the odd, contorted positions Ebersole has placed her in so that her body will yield up the shadowy secret it has been harboring.

The shading is still there, a little more definite this time. "You can clearly see the upper lobe on this one," says Ebersole, not a little proud of his photography. "See this line, it's pretty well articulated. No wonder you couldn't outline it on palpation; it's just too well hidden."

Bairstow looks numbly at the film. This is the moment he's been dreading, the clearer plate showing more precise contours of the process giving June distress. He places his finger on the film and traces the shadow.

"What do you think?" Ebersole asks after a minute. "Surgery or radiation or both."

Bairstow hesitates, then shakes his head: his normal thought processes are not progressing smoothly. "I don't know. I'll have to discuss it with the patient--June--and Potter. We'll see. What do you think, Max?"

Ebersoles stares at the films, his head beside Bairstow's as he compares them. Thank God, Bairstow thinks, that the smell of his lilac cologne has dissipated. "We'll need a CAT scan, I'd say. Then maybe we can wash out some cells for analysis."

Bairstow nods. What Ebersole is suggesting he'll go along with: the CAT scan will delineate, layer by layer, what June is harboring in the lung area. Later they will try surgically to free a few cells if at all possible. Bairstow had not realized how tough, just how really diffficult, nerve-racking and draining, it will be to go through this process when one is involved so emotionally. It is shattering, this play-by-play response to the body's malfunction, move and counter-move, like a deadly chess game.

"You're sure you want to see the other films?" Ebersole asks, the expression on his face conveying--"or have you seen enough for this day?"

When Bairstow nods, Ebersole flips the others onto the screen, one after the other: a broken leg on the first, question of gallstones in the neck of the bladder, question of bone chips in the spine on a third. All will require Bairstow's attention sooner or later.

"You'll be busy," says Ebersole.

"Yes." It's the least of Bairstow's problems right now, that he'll be busy.

"You have patients this afternoon, Ben?" Ebersole prods, assessing Bairstow's day with genuine interest.

Somehow, Bairstow feels, there's comfort in it. "A few house patients. Then I'm going home."

"You'll tell Mrs. Potter? You don't want me to report it?"

"I'll tell her, Max. June will have to tell Potter herself. She's the patient, after all. She can handle very well...whatever is involved."

"I'm sure, Bairstow." Ebersole seems to be asking another question--Bairstow can see it in his eyes:--whether he, Bairstow, can handle it.

Bairstow doesn't answer, he picks up his jacket and turns away from the screen, his face becoming darker as the light, like an eclipse, leaves it. He has no answer to Ebersole's question, nor does he wish to dwell on it. He takes the elevator to the main part of the hospital where the wards are located to see his patients, not having the energy to climb the stairs. In the company of one of the surgical nurses on duty, Joanne Shay, he begins at one end of the ward and works his way systematically down the corridor, percussing, palpating, prescribing. In an hour he is finished. For another thirty minutes he annotates the charts, then writes discharge notes on the two patients who are to leave. "Call me if you need me," Bairstow tells the nurse. "I'll have my cellphone." He smiles briefly. "I won't try to get away."

"Didn't think you would," says Joanne with a grin. He plucks the phone from a drawer where it resides in the surgical station, a drawer which also houses surgical tape and scissors, a broken pair of clamps, an ancient issue of the AMA journal, tongue depressors and a used tea bag. One of these days, Bairtow thinks, someone will clean out that drawer, but he's not about to do it today.

He starts home, following the usual route, but somehow finds himself making a right turn instead of a left, and then another to the right, getting closer to Potter's place all the time. But someone has to tell June about Ebersole's findings, he's promised--or so he tells himself. No, says another voice just as clearly, you intended to do this all the time. Barsamian, the psychologist: Bairstow can hear him very well right now--would click his tongue, finger his moustache, and eye him triumphantly as if to say, I told you so, Freud lives. But he *has* promised June, she shouldn't wait any longer in limbo as she must be doing now. But, he wonders, what on earth is kindness: is it to give her a few more minutes or hours of peace, or to present to her these indications of her fate as soon as possible so as to lessen the period of her uncertainty? Can she handle it, can anyone? But wasn't that what June had said about Amanda, that she should be allowed the freedom to face her own destiny? What June was asserting was that she could face her own, too; but can she really when the chips are down, when that shadow is so closely revealed? And is Amanda really able to avoid those crippling pitfalls of youth which have incapacitated so many children of this generation?

Probably, thinks Bairstow, but he'll be here for both Amanda and June just in case they aren't as strong as they think they are. For he is coming to find that he isn't as invulnerable as he'd thought *he* was, either. It's terrible to find that one is subject to all the ravages he's seen in others, those flaws that he, as a doctor and healer, had thought he was impervious to. All right, he'll try to present as much invincibility as he can manage, to give courage to June and a certain amount of starch to Amanda, although perhaps Amanda needs less starch and merely a good old-fashioned talking-to. He wonders what Barsamian would think of *that*! Or June. Amanda has spunk and is as stubborn as he is, that's the problem. But how is she using it, that's also the problem. To thwart her parents? Or thumb her nose at common sense? To break the law? But that's pure utter idiocy, and somewhere along the line, if Bairstow can keep his wits about himself and his temper under control, she must be reeled in or assisted or cajoled or even threatened with the folly of it. He doesn't want her to destroy herself in this rebellion--and himself and Miriam as well.

Bairstow is turning the corner to June's house--he can see it now, the high glass windows reflecting the muted light of this wan day, a gathering of pewter dullness and pale tarnish. He hasn't even called to see if she is home, but he feels that she will be there; perhaps he's acquiring a second sense about things after all, who knows? But he senses her presence somehow and turns at the drive almost as if summoned.

She answers the door; she's dressed in a simple dressing gown, long and sapphire blue, falling from her breasts to the floor in a single flowing line. About her throat is a single strand of small milky pearls which almost blend with the color and texture of her skin. She steps back to let him enter. "Somehow I knew you'd come," she says. "I think

I expected you. You see, I even dressed; until a half-hour ago I was wearing my paint clothes."

Bairstow enters the foyer, and she takes his jacket. He is again impressed with the beauty of this house, with the muted light which comes in from the high windows, and the long drapes, partly open, which frame them.

"When do you expect Potter back?" Bairstow asks. It will be of help to her, he thinks, if Potter is here after he leaves.

"I don't know—tomorrow, I think. Why? Are you afraid you'll see him, Ben, or is it that you want to talk to him?"

He steps back. "Afraid to see Potter? You know me better than that, June. I wouldn't have come here if I were afraid to see him, and if I'd wanted to see him I'd have called."

"Good. Then you wanted to see me. Come in, Ben. I wanted to see you, too, but you must know that already. I fear, however, that this isn't entirely a social call." She leads him slowly into the living room, into the sunken section where she places a cushion behind her back and her feet along the length of the couch. At her nod, he shifts a pillow and sits opposite.

Bairstow leans forward to see her face in the semi-light of the room. "How do you know why I've come, June?"

"Because you've read the X-rays, my dear. And now you've come to tell me what you've found."

Is it so obvious? Bairstow wonders. He'd at least wanted to shield her from the blow, to lead her into it gradually.

"And," she goes on, "it isn't so promising, is it, or you'd be full of smiles? I think I can see through you a little by now. Isn't that marvelous? Well, perhaps you'd better tell me right out what they showed, because I was never very good at mysteries."

Bairstow nods solemnly and places one fist inside the palm of the other hand. "I've been with Ebersole, June. There's something on the film, but the nature of it still eludes us. He thinks we should try a CAT scan, to define it more closely. I thought I'd tell you myself, since Potter is away, and besides, you indicated that you wanted to know right away. I...wish I could tell you something more positive, I honestly wish I could."

When he looks at June, her face is somber, but her eyes are fixed unflinchingly on his.

"Thank you, Ben. You were...wonderful to come all the way over here, you could have merely telephoned. But I knew you would, isn't that interesting? If only all doctors were as thoughtful as you."

Bairstow studies her face and wonders if she's run into some pretty bad doctors in the past or is simply complimenting him. And into what category does Potter fall in her scheme of things, in her evaluation of the profession?

"I want you to know," Bairstow continues, "that I'm here always, and if I can help you, I will. I've been through this with some of my patients...not so personally, of course, I'm sorry to say that. Perhaps I haven't felt enough for them, and I'm at fault for that. But I care about you and what you're going through, and maybe that's enough for now."

She swings her legs from the couch and comes to sit beside him, almost touching his shoulder. "I've felt your kindness and your concern since we met, Ben. I think you've considered yourself to be responsible for your entire world, but you aren't, you know. You're not responsible for me. But your consideration means everything. I think that if you care, I'll make it no matter what happens. And if you don't care, I won't. It's as simple as that."

Bairstow instinctively leans forward to touch her cheek, the most natural gesture in the world. Her hand is on the back of his head, and she presses herself against him. "You're the most decent man I've met in a long while," she murmurs, "maybe forever. Thank you, my dear, for your strength."

"I care about you, I do, I want you to know that. Perhaps I shouldn't, but I do. I want to help you any way I can."

Her arms tighten about him, as if their control is almost involuntary. "I'm causing you all kinds of difficulty..."

"Difficulty?" He guesses immediately what she means. "No, June. I know that there are problems between you and Potter, I don't even want to know what they are. But I admire you enormously, you've already saved my life this day with Amanda."

They're silent for a moment, Bairstow's arm about her shoulders, protectively. It's a moment of peace and fullness, a trusting interval he thought would never happen again in his life, an interlude full of implication and wonder. June moves against him. "Would you like to sleep with me, Ben?" she asks. "I mean, I don't want to entice you this way, then back away."

Bairstow can smell the sweet scent of her hair, soft beneath his chin. He feels heady with the intoxication of her nearness, but this doesn't seem the place nor the time to him. It isn't right. "Perhaps, but not now, June. Just because I'm concerned about you is no reason for you to show me gratitude I don't deserve."

She stirs beside him, pulling herself upright. "I wouldn't do that... ever. I'd only be with you if that's what you wanted and what I wanted. I virtually decided that the last time I saw you in this house. It wasn't very long ago, only a few days, but somehow it seems like light years, like eons..."

Bairstow strokes her cheek again. "How much of this will you tell Potter?'"

"You mean about...whatever it is that seems to have invaded my body?"

"That, too."

"Nothing about the first, for now, and everything about the second. He is my husband and should know what threatens my health because it affects him. About you and me: the fact that you are my friend makes me happy; it has nothing to do with Jeff. Yet maybe someday I'll tell him, I don't know. He knows I admire you. And sometimes one needs to do the things necessary for one's happiness..and perhaps even for one's survival."

Whatever passes between Potter and June must be devastating, Bairstow thinks, for such spaces to have come between them. If it's

only simple incompatibility in a marriage, even that can be grievous
enough.

"And will you tell Miriam?" June asks. "You are close to her?"

"I love her, yes, and I'd never hurt her, not ever. But for some reason,
my life is at a point of crisis, and she knows it as well as I. I don't think
Miriam can help me, much as she tries. It has to do with Amanda, and
the boys, and my professional life."

"Quite a scope," says June. "Don't you think that people reevaluate
themselves at intervals in their lives, to sort of gird themselves for what
comes next?"

"I suppose. Yes, I think they do."

"Well, I understand because that's what I'm doing: going down for
the count. You see, my brother was a boxer in college, and I know what
it means. But I intend to get up slugging again when I decide how to
handle this temporary knockdown."

It amuses Bairstow to think of June comparing herself to a boxer in
a ring; yet he can see the logic of what she's saying. She *has* had a blow,
and when she recovers from the shock of it, she will make her own way
once again. Perhaps that is the best way, Bairstow thinks; he will have
served his purpose and hers. Yet he is not sure when all is over how *he*
will react emotionally, and what this involvement will do to his inner
strength and sense of well-being. But you don't know anything about
yourself until you venture out in a new direction, Bairstow decides. For
better or worse.

June leans forward. "Ben, I love you for coming here today. It must
have been torture for you, pure hell, to tell me news I didn't want to
hear. I thank you for that, dear friend. Jeff will, too, when I tell him."

"I hope he comes back soon. It's not easy to be alone when you face
a crisis."

"Sometimes it's better, honestly. My best moments are when I'm by
myself, I think. Then I'm full of great courage and resolve. It's when I'm
surrounded by people that I discover what a weakling I really am."

"There's always strength in having your friends and family around
you, June. Incidentally, I think you have admirable strength."

"Thanks, Ben. But it depends on the family and friends. Sometimes family can be worse than anyone. And friends may be wonderful. But you can rely on yourself most of all when things get really bad. I mean, sometimes there's no choice, and you find that you can make it when you didn't think you could."

"Of course. What was your father like, June? Independent and resourceful? He was very much a pioneer in our field, but I know nothing about him."

She rests her chin on her hand. "I...I guess he's viewed that way by his colleagues. Terrible as if sounds, I never understood him well enough to know. I...I don't think he ever trusted anyone, isn't that terrible? He considered it a weakness to invest any emotional weight in another. Somehow he didn't need us. I've even envied that quality, but it wouldn't work for me. I couldn't take the isolation, nor the total confidence he must have placed on his own worth."

Bairstow can picture June's father now: a solemn, dignified, tall man with graying hair who conducted the most significant hospital rounds of Bairstow's career, but who inspired awe and even fear, in his students.

"The worst regret I have," June is continuing, "is that I never made it with him. I told you. I was always sickly with hay fever, then I broke my leg, and continually ran into poison ivy. All the miserable kid things."

"But wasn't your mother sympathetic?"

"Yes. But the one I wanted to please was my father, isn't that absurd? And I was merely incidental to his life. Big heart surgeons don't notice when their kids have chicken pox, do they?"

June is still leaning against his shoulder, and he can feel her agitation, a small quaking like a sapling in a windstorm. "Some do," he says, "it depends on the man. Undoubtedly it was his loss. It's true, his generation--and mine a little, too--didn't have time for such things. But in a way I admire men like your father: somehow they were all bigger than life, as if refracted in a prism, and not like ordinary mortals at all."

"But they *are* merely mortal, Ben. I feel the pathos of that mystique. I'm a victim of it. Yet I can't tell you how much I loved my father...how I admired him. He loved me, too; we simply couldn't communicate. Jeff is the same way in some respects: isn't it ironic, what the psychiatrists say, that sometimes you marry your own father? Faced with what's ahead, I don't know if I can depend on Jeff for much support. Oh, he'll be kind, but I can't draw on his strength."

"But Potter has...potential, June. I suspect he's got flexibility in ways your father didn't. He may surprise you. And you're resourceful—a talented artist as well as a friendly, open person, at least with me. Maybe we're all pretty enclosed in ways I wish we weren't."

She cradles her chin in her hand, then nods and smiles. "I think you're right, Ben. I've never talked to anyone like this before. Do you mind when I run on this way?"

"Of course not. I told you, that's what I'm here for."

"You're not angry or anything?"

"Why on earth would I be angry? You're a fascinating, delightful woman. I could never be angry with you."

He can hear her intake of breath. "Thank you, Ben. You'll come again soon?" He turns to kiss her lightly on the forehead, instead takes her into his arms and holds her against his chest. "Soon."

"Good. You know, I think I love you a little. I'll follow whatever you and Dr. Ebersole decide...and Jeff, of course."

He leaves knowing that the ultimate decision belongs to June and Jeff—but he also knows that he has the primary medical responsibility because she is his patient. He feels the weight of that responsibility as he returns to the hospital.

CHAPTER ELEVEN

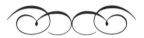

Amanda is already home: Bairstow can see her car, a small blue Volkswagen, parked in the bushes beyond the driveway. He and Miriam gave it to her when she left for prep school, so that she could return home on the theory that she might be homesick and want to visit them or her friends. Actually, this is the first time she's been home, to his knowledge. So much for homesickness, Bairstow thinks.

Inside, he finds Miriam writing letters in the alcove off the kitchen: it is her favorite place in the entire house. "Since you turned the living room into a tomb," Miriam told him once--in the days before she filled part of it with her favorite piece of furniture, her mother's grand piano--"this is the only place I feel comfortable." Even now it's true that more often than not when she's home alone, she uses the kitchen and the small room beyond as the hub of her activities, writing letters, visiting with friends, even reading correspondence and books in close proximity to the stove and refrigerator on one side and the sliding doors to the patio and grassy area where Bairstow keeps his garden chair on the other. Amanda is nowhere to be seen.

Bairstow gives her a kiss on the forehead. "You've had a long day," says Miriam, peering at him over her reading glasses. "Can't you sit down?"

"I can't. I feel restless."

She continues to look at him appraisingly. "Did you know that Amanda's home? She says she's home for the weekend. She has to check in with the court on Monday."

"I saw her car." Bairstow is about to tell her that he saw Amanda at the restaurant, but omits the fact. He can feel a pang from the omission, but puts it aside for now.

"Are you covering for Potter this weekend?" Miriam can see the cellphone hooked to his belt; if he were free, he'd have left it in that drawer at the hospital.

"Yes. He's off at some damned bicycle race."

Miriam looks at him quickly again: she's never known him to criticize Potter so sharply. She purses her lips and says nothing.

"What's Amanda doing?" Bairstow asks. "Where is she?"

"In her room. She's got her door locked. I tried to talk to her but she won't open up. Bairstow, will you talk to her? She can't spend the entire weekend cooped up."

Bairstow looks at his wife with surprise and shakes his head. "Well, if that's where she wants to be, I'm not going to dissuade her. Besides, if she won't come out for you, I'm damned sure she won't come out for me."

"But we can try. I think she spent her entire junior year of high school locked up in that room. I can't understand why her silent treatment has to go on forever, can you? My Lord, what does one do with children like that? It's as if we've become virtually untouchable."

Bairstow remembers the attempts before to reach Amanda, which usually ended in mutual hostility and recriminations. They left him feeling inadequate and angry. Usually he solved his feelings by going back to work: there were always patients who needed him. Miriam was never able to cope any better than he was, yet she didn't have the escape hatch he did.

"I'll try to talk to her, Miriam, but that's never helped much before. She'll call me names, I'll get angry, and what good is that?" Besides, after the confrontation at the restaurant he feels that such an unpleasant result is virtually assured.

"Then *don't* get angry, Bairstow. You can control yourself, can't you? You're the adult, after all."

"Well, she isn't exactly a child anymore, either." These women, Bairstow thinks, judge me to be some kind of superman, capable of handling all things. But the fact is, he feels inadequate to handle this despite June's good words and Miriam's plea. Damn it, if Amanda *did* steal something, she can take care of it herself and be her own keeper, as June suggested, but talking to her is another thing. Yet he dutifully marches up the stairs, standing before Amanda's door as if to gain courage and resolve. Then he raps against the wood with his knuckles, not too forcefully as to appear insistent, but sufficiently firm to sound as if he means it. So ridiculous, Bairstow thinks, worrying about how to knock on your own daughter's door. Actually, he'd like to beat the thing down and scare the hell out of her for once, if for no other reason than to call attention to the fact that he feels equally left out of her life.

For a moment there's no answer. Bairstow knocks again: maybe she's asleep. Then he hears a faint stirring; she's awake all right. "Who is it?" Amanda asks in a tired, bored voice.

"Your father. Open up, Amanda, I'd like to talk to you."

"About what?"

"Come on, I'm not going to stand out here in this hall talking to myself."

To his surprise, he can hear her reluctant footsteps approaching across the room. Then a key turns in the lock. The door opens to reveal Amanda dressed in jeans and an old sweater; she's changed from the dress she'd worn so suggestively earlier at the restaurant. Undoubtedly by now it's hanging again in her mother's closet. "What do you want?" she asks.

"May I come in, Amanda?"

Bairstow knows that Amanda is not only surprised to find him here, but a little nonplussed as well. He also notes that her face is washed of the lipstick and purple eye-tint she'd used to heighten her color. Just now, Bairstow thinks, she looks almost like a little girl in the gentle contour of her face and the uncertain way she holds her head. It's a shame, he thinks, a damned shame that all this is happening.

"I was surprised to see you earlier," Bairstow says, opening tentatively. "I'm afraid it really caught me by surprise."

"I bet it did," Amanda counters. "Who is that woman you were with?"

Immediately something in Bairstow's viceral being begins to contract. "To begin with, it's none of your business. I might ask you the same."

"Well, isn't that what you intend to do? You're here to give me a hard time, to grill me..."

Bairstow takes a deep breath, fighting for control. "I don't know what I'm here for, to tell you the truth. I guess I wanted to say hello. I behaved pretty badly at the restaurant..."

For a moment Amanda is silent, frowning at him. "Well, he's just a friend and you needn't get bent about it. He isn't going to carry your little girl off, you know."

"I didn't suppose he was. I was simply astonished...to run into you that way."

"Because it was such a ritzy place? You thought only doctors could eat in such fancy places?"

Bairstow rakes his fingers through his hair. As usual, their discussion is getting nowhere. What on God's earth had he and Miriam done to deserve this treatment? He turns to leave, his eyes sweeping across the shelves of stuffed animals, the ruffled bedspreads on the twin beds, the shelves of books and walls of memorabilia including a bank of pictures in frames of people he doesn't know. At least Amanda cares for someone and something even if it isn't us, he's thinking. Maybe that's enough. Let her go, June said, but it's so darned hard. But just maybe that's what he's been wanting to do for months, even years, and hasn't known how. It's true that at the age of consent one is responsible for one's self... within reason. Lord knows the twins manage better than Amanda: they're always out playing soccer, or camping, or doing something with their friends with enthusiasm and without a peep of complaint.

But Amanda is different. He simply can't dismiss her like this. "You'll be down later for dinner?"

Amanda shakes her head. "I'm going out."

"Well, have a good evening." I'll miss you, he almost says.

Amanda stares at him as if she's expecting him to stop her, to exert parental authority; her lips are tight with the retort she'd been about to make. "You still didn't say who you were out with," she says. "Who was that lady?"

Bairstow, who's been about to leave, turns back to face her. Perhaps he should feel angry, he thinks--Lord knows, he was angry earlier. But this time he's only sad. "Come off it, Amanda," he says. "Why don't you stop acting like a...damned...little...baby?" Then he turns again and walks slowly back down the stairs.

"You talked to her?" Miriam asks. She's standing at the kitchen counter, right where he left her, and Bairstow knows she hasn't been reading her book, or sewing, or writing shopping lists; she's been suffering, waiting for voices to be raised which would indicate verbal struggle between her child and spouse. It's something which Miriam has never been able to stand, the sounds of strife. Perhaps, thinks Bairstow, she's been programmed for tranquility as I've been for insensitivity. The "tall, silent type," he thinks, what a fraud. But no worse than "peace and quiet", her dictum for family living. She's right, it's a wonderful goal--but maybe I should have screamed a lot and she should have cried more and things might have gone better.

"I *tried* to talk to her," Bairstow corrects Mirium. "She interrogated her wayward father, showing him the error of his ways, then announced she was leaving--oh, not for good, but for the evening. I'm sure she'll be ravenous for breakfast. I guess our room and board still pass muster, but our company doesn't."

Miriam continues to stand stiffly at the kitchen counter, slicing carrots. "I wish you two could get along," she says. "No, I wish I could get along with her. I never seem to say anything right." She looks as if she might cry. "I wish I knew what I did wrong. The parole officer wants us to come with Amanda to the hearing, and I know I won't be able to keep a stiff upper lip, I just know it."

"Why do we have to go?"

"As her guardians, for support..." She dries her eyes on a kitchen towel. "Bairstow, I cried my way through the last hearing, even though it took less than ten minutes, and I can't face it again. I can't control myself so how am I supposed to give guidance to her..."

Bairstow leans toward her; he's been resting his frame on the other end of the counter. "Miriam, we aren't going to the conference with the parole officer, either of us."

"We're not...?"

"What Amanda got herself into she can get out of...by herself. Not five minutes ago she gave me the boot. Well, it works both ways. Why does anyone have to put up with that sort of thing, including--and maybe especially--your own offspring? As far as I'm concerned I'll do what's necessary to keep her going, but not a bit more. When she began stealing, she went out on her own. Why, you ought to see," Bairstow begins, on the verge of telling her about the dress Amanda had filched for the luncheon, then thinks better of it, adding "What do other parents I've read about do with their kids who steal?" and finishes lamely but firmly, "They throw them right out of the house. It's pretty grim, but they do it just the same."

"But she's only eighteen, Ben. You can't leave a child of eighteen..."

Bairstow feels some pangs, seeing Miriam so dejected. "I'm not advocating abandoning her, Miriam. I love her as much as you do. But why doesn't she shape up? I can't understand it. Don't girls of eighteen have responsibilities toward those around them? Doesn't she care at all that we feed and clothe her? Extremely well, I might add. Will we always be villains in her head?"

"She *cares*, Bairstow, but you make it sound so stark. We *do* love her, you just said it, and I ache for her sometimes."

Bairstow comes across to Miriam and kisses her on the cheek. "Mimi, when the boys come home, let's go out for a hamburg. I don't want to sit around here feeling guilty about Amanda. I want to do something different."

"A hamburg? I didn't think you *liked* hamburgs. 'All that fat and bread,' and that's an exact quote."

"Must you repeat my weaker moments to me?"

"And the boys won't be home for another hour. Little League practice..."

"Then let's wait. I want to dig out my recent journals, anyway, for anything I can find on tumors of the ventral area."

"That sounds fine, Bairstow, but I can't figure out what's got into you lately."

What's important, Bairstow is thinking, is that I've got to get hold of myself if I'm going to be any good for anyone else, Amanda and June included. Maybe I've never learned to care sufficiently before—it takes some kind of specal skills. What I don't have is the answer to caring on one hand and detachment on the other. But I know I can't tolerate any longer those who don't at least try to join the human race, even if I'm one of them, and the other is my own daughter.

He pulls out his journals from a shelf in the living room, a stack of them, half of which he's read thoroughly, the others only partially and, in the third stack, they've not even been removed from their jackets. He simply hasn't had time to get to them, yet he always enjoys them. Occasionally he stops to admire the garish advertisements depicting the organs of the body in bright shades of red and blue--because they're actually ingenious and well-done; yet they appall laymen, and patients in the waiting room complain so he doesn't mix them with his popular magazines. Yet those overlays illustrating the body's structure are works of art, leaving one breathless at the skill required to draw them. Most of the people who were responsible for publishing them, he's sure, never saw the interior of the body--the plates were planned and produced in some advertising agency far removed from pulsing blood and decrepit ganglia. But they are nevertheless awesome in their precision: this artery goes there, in that bright red area, and that vein there, in the blue one, and it somehow appears so satisfyingly bright, neat and easy that Bairstow wishes it really *did* appear like that. Looking at the ads, one can merely admire the skill of it all.

Bairstow is looking for an article he'd seen a month--or was it two months ago?--describing the latest cures for cancer, including a learned discussion of methods of proceeding with lung lesions. He remembers it vaguely, but now it's urgent that he find it. He's determined to put his hand on it. Of course, he can call experts in the field, but he wants to peruse this article first. He wants to understand the palpable effects of chemotherapy on chest lesions, to know precisely where the oncologists stand even though nothing has been decided about June. But somehow it helps him to be reading rather than merely speculating about the problem. Like other scientists, he has a lifelong trust in basic research: if the best journals report from the oncologists that there's hope, he'll pretty much believe it. Bairstow has tried, on his own, alternative cures and radical procedures, and some of them have worked, so he knows perfectly well that all change and cures don't emanate from medical centers or even from researchers, but from doctors like him who work in the field and spark most progress in his specialty. So where, he wonders, is that journal?

It takes him 15 minutes before he finally lays his hand on the text he's been seeking, accompanied by graphs and charts embedded in the data. On the way he uncovers several others he intends to look over eventually, when he has time.

He carries the scotch and water he'd poured for himself to the cavernous leather chair situated by the window, where he does serious reading. At least if no one else wants to use this place, he thinks, I will. He flips up the foot section so that he's reclining like one of his own patients. He can feel his arteries slow and his pulses ease. This, he thinks fatalistically, is probably the place where I'll have a heart attack one day--and the irony of the fact makes him chuckle, that the body could rebel not under stress but under relaxation. Few surgeons he knows have succumbed at the operating table; they've met their demise loafing. At least it's a more convenient way to go, he thinks--I'd hate to leave some poor guy under anesthesia while I expire under the table. Of course, the assisting surgeon would take over, but it would be damned awkward for the poor guy with two inert bodies to cope with.

The article isn't long but the researchers have done their work well. He vaguely knows one of the men who co-signed the article, a respected thoracic surgeon who gave a closed-circuit lecture to his group at a medical meeting he'd attended three or four years ago. It all boils down to what Bairstow already knows: if there's a mass, it's best to remove it, then use chemotherapy. Of course, it depends on the mass, on what one finds from X-ray and other tests. All this has happened so fast that it makes one's head spin. Bairstow has always felt so sure, so confident of his skills before, but now he doesn't know anymore. A week ago he could have given a considered judgment on precisely what should happen in June's case, his mind functioning smoothly and surely. Yet now he finds himself wavering ever so slightly in indecision and uncertainty, second-guessing his own decisions. He's never had this feeling of helplessness before, but he can feel it now, formless but palpable, making him profoundly uneasy.

He places his glass on the table beside him, raises his chair to upright, then carries into the kitchen the journal folded back to the article. He sits on one of the stools, placing the issue before him on the counter. Miriam looks up, not speaking, waiting for her husband to begin. She's a woman long used to Bairstow's habits, and she reads his moods better even than do the nurses at the hospital.

"I'm afraid that June Potter has cancer," he says simply. He suddenly feels drained and can't find the energy to explain, to elucidate, to amplify. But the bald statement itself sends out its own shock waves.

Miriam turns to look at him. For a moment she, too, is at a loss for words. "My God," she asks, "is it serious? Where is it situated?"

Bairstow moves his hand to his own chest. "Thorax. Shadows on X-ray. I've seen too many of them not to know. God, I wish I didn't."

Miriam hasn't moved; it's as if the two of them are held in place by an exterior force. "Does her husband know?" she asks.

Bairstow shakes his head. "I can't tell him if she doesn't give me permission. It's her business to tell Potter. Pretty tough, though, if she doesn't. I can't imagine operating every day with the man and knowing something like that about his wife that he doesn't know. But she'll tell him, I'm sure of it. He takes these damned weekends and...leaves her to cope.

"It's really a shame, Ben."

Bairstow nods. "Well, call me when the twins come back." He picks up the journal and returns to the living room, where he drops it on the pile and relaxes again in the chair, there to nurse along the rest of his scotch, which is now turning watery. He sits back and contemplates the ceiling. The house is quiet. Somewhere upstairs his daughter sulks, but down here the silence and approaching dark keep him and Miriam away from her, yet all three separate into their distinct worlds. Still, he's always wanted this, his private life, and the distance he maintains from those about himself. His space is inviolable. Miriam knows it--she has her space, too--and his children know it. Even Amanda upstairs knows the borders...and how to cross them if she wants to be a little savage.

Bairstow thinks about it a moment, that space, and Amanda...and June. He's breached a border to June, let down one of his guards. How far she'll come in he doesn't know. There's a penalty about it for him, though: he's sacrificed a little of his turf. With the loss of his valued distance has seeped away some of his detachment and independence. That's the sanction, and Bairstow doesn't know where it will end. It's almost as if in some ways June's a daughter of his middle years, but not quite. She's not a daughter, and far from a wife, and not exactly a mere friend, either. She's in a category of her own.

He thinks of the things June said about Amanda--about allowing the girl her own space, and says under his breath, as if addressing his daughter, "All right, kiddo, now you've got it, what are you going to do with it?" But he doesn't entirely agree with June, either. Amanda is *his* daughter, after all, and that makes all the difference.

Bairstow hasn't an idea how it will turn out, or what use his daughter will make of her life when he and Miriam pass on. Will she straighten out, will she go her own way on more reliable pathways than those she's sought out this far? Or will she join a host of bratty children such as he's seen in the past, some in the homes of his own colleagues? Or will she turn to something stronger; maybe some good stock still remains in the old family tree. He became a doctor, after all, which isn't so bad. He smiles to himself in the dark; so maybe there's something left somewhere in the old hybrid.

It isn't funny, Bairstow is thinking, I've been drinking too damned much scotch. Besides, a sobering thought has just crept into his brain: Amanda never told Miriam that he'd taken June to lunch. Why didn't she? Was she trying to protect her errant father through some sort of misguided family solidarity? Is he really an errant father? He hopes to God he isn't. All his life he's taken responsibility for others in what he feels is the best way he knows. He hasn't thought about it much, he's just done it. Where could anything he's done have gone so wrong?

It couldn't have. This is an absurd conjecture. He's a success by most standards, he's got a wonderful family. Well, it's probably about the same as everyone else's, but to him it's the best. Even that young woman upstairs: if she'd straighten out she'd find out how much good stuff has been put into her without her knowing it or having anything to do with it; and if she started giving some of it back to others, she'd do herself and everyone else a favor. Yet maybe he should start examining himself more, on the assumption that Amanda didn't get that way by herself. Is he at fault somehow? His feelings stirring ever so tentatively make him uncomfortable.

He feels himself growing relaxed and drowsy--it's been a tough day. It's always a tough day in his business, but he'd accepted that a long time ago, and it's suited his temperament. As a kid, he'd had more energy than anyone else around. He'd never been able to understand weak kids, quiet kids--yet he'd gone into the business of caring for those less fortunate, who came to him not in strength but in weakness. He's pleased about that even if he doesn't quite understand it.

And where did that leave June? Lord knows, she wasn't weak. Probably she's stronger than I am, Bairstow thinks. She understands things about Amanda I can't...and about other matters as well. Maybe she knows me better than I know myself. I'd probably collapse if I had something growing inside me that might sap my strength and shorten my life. I'd probably go crazy or end it all. Yes, that's probably exactly what I'd do if I didn't have the guts to tough it out.

How long do I have to sit around here waiting for those kids at Little League, he thinks a little testily. What's that coach up to, anyway, that he wants to keep my kids up half the night? Doesn't he understand that they eat like other people, and so do their parents?

To his surprise, just as he's thinking the words, the back door slams and he can hear the twins falling into the kitchen the way they always do, in a sort of controlled crash, dragging books, bats, belongings and themselves through the single door at the same minute.

He welcomes the change, to get out of this chair, out of this room, out of his mood. He even savors the thought of a hamburger. I don't know what's wrong with me, he thinks, but I'll go along with it and see what happens. I'll think about June and Amanda later.

CHAPTER TWELVE

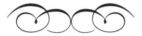

The twins are built tall like Bairstow, but both look like their mother, dark and slim, though she's widened about the middle after having brought three children into the world. Bairstow is glad they resemble Miriam--she's a good-looking woman. Amanda looks like him: reddish hair which she touches up, according to Miriam, while to his chagrin his is graying around the temples. All have firm chins (Amanda's can be pugnacious sometimes), hazel eyes which appear almost blue, and stand tall as young trees. Bairstow, however, has developed a slight slouch which he attributes to hours bent over the operating table. Once Amanda had a quick, easy, agreeable smile but he hasn't seen it in months. She's mostly downcast or sometimes even sullen. But he isn't a big smiler, either—he's got too much on his mind.

When it seems as though the boys are at last settling down, having passed through the first surge of explosive energy at arriving home, he walks slowly into the kitchen. "Hi, Dad," yells Pete, the most ebullient of the two. "Mom says we're heading out to dinner." It's almost a question, because usually the last thing in the world Bairstow wants to do after a busy day is go out to dinner. Norman pauses in mid-stride to hear if his mother had been hearing right when Bairstow had suggested such a thing.

"How's it sound to you?" asks Bairstow, pursuing the point. "Would you fellows rather have a hamburg or a pizza?" Maybe they'll not think I'm such an old fogy after all, he thinks--but then, relenting, he knows they don't think such a thing at all. He's merely a little down on himself right now.

"Pizza," yells Norman. "With pepperoni...and mushrooms...and the works."

"Hamburgs," calls Pete. "With onions, and ketchup, and cheese."

A frontal assault. He can see Miriam smiling, wondering how he's going to handle the insurrection. "Then I get the veto," he says. "Hamburgs it is. I haven't had one in...weeks."

Norman peers at him quizzically, stuffing his hands into his pockets. "But it isn't fair. How come *you* get the veto?"

"Easy," answers Bairstow. "Because I'm paying for it, that's why I've got the veto. Are you guys ready to go?"

Pete shakes his head. "Don't you give a guy time to go pee?" He wiggles around inside his pants as if to demonstrate the urgency of his plight.

"Peter Bairstow!" exclaims Miriam. "Can't you refrain from saying such things out loud?"

It hits Bairstow as funny: it's better that they bellow about their private functions here at home than elsewhere, isn't it? Besides, his son's references to his excretory functions are tame compared to what he hears during any ten-minute period in the hospital. He glances at Miriam and realizes that she's trying hard not to laugh and that she's not half as provoked as she'd sounded.

Pete bounds across the kitchen, on a direct path to the downstairs bathroom. Norman grins, as if not quite believing what he's just seen. He's a quieter child, more like Bairstow even if he doesn't carry the paternal family resemblance. "How come you don't need to pee?" Bairstow asks Norman. "You've got the capacity of a camel?"

"Peed in the bushes," says Norman in a matter-of-fact voice. "Else I never would'a made it, either."

Miriam's eyebrows rise an inch, but she only glances at Bairstow—he's doing so well, she seems to be thinking, that he might as well carry the ball. But she wonders what bush Norman had used, hoping it wasn't one of the new, young arborvitae beside the door that Bairstow has just put in this year. Of course, they'll find out soon enough anyway, when the leaves begin to wither and turn brown.

"We'll take the truck," says Bairstow in a sudden decision. "Your mother and I will be right out."

This time Norman stops dead in his tracks. "You mean it? The truck?"

It's an old truck that Bairstow had bought for a thousand bucks from a neighbor who'd been about to scrap it. It's been useful to drag equipment around, to move bushes, stones and balled trees from one side of the property to the other, and to tow a small boat to the lake. Often he's let the boys ride in the back, but he'd never suggested they could go into town before. Now, he thinks, I'm glad I paid that extra thousand bucks to keep the damn thing in working order.

Miriam, with an amused look in her eye, today seems perfectly content, Bairstow thinks, to ride up front in the cab which has been shorn of every vestige of upholstery which had at one time undoubtedly graced the seats. Bairstow, when he bought the truck from the neighbor, purchased cushions from a dealer to place loosely over the exposed springs--but now even they are insufficiently comfortable to allow one decent dignity in traveling very far. All in all, it isn't a bad piece of machinery, though, and if it adds to the boys' fun and doesn't detract from Miriam's, why not use the old vehicle?

Behind them, the boys sit in the enclosed truckbed, chatting amiably as if this were the most natural thing in the world. Of course, we do this all the time, they seem to be implying. "We ride around in this truck day in, day out." If there were a vote, Bairstow knows, they'd take the truck over the Lexus any day. This is the life, what a lark!

It *is* a lark, the whole thing. Bairstow knows it will end, but for now it's one of the more spontaneous things they've done in a while. They'll remember it, Bairstow thinks, and I don't want to forget it. It's high time they had some fun.

Miriam, too, is in the spirit of the thing: the smile on her face seems to say, "I don't know why we're doing this, but I'll go along with it." No--Bairstow looks closer--she's really enjoying it. It's as if she scented the air and found it perfectly appropriate to slander family decorum. She glances over at him in a congratulatory way, virtually tipping her hat to her husband's ingenuousness and aplomb. Yes, for some reason Bairstow does feel at ease and lighthearted for the first time in days. He feels a diminution of pressure, a cessation of pain, a lightening of the entire body mass and a shift in its chemistry...as if, by taking a new tack, one can elude concern. It seems so simple, so elementary. He sits at the wheel of the truck, directing the retooled, formerly rusting machinery, out the drive and into the stream of traffic, turning to the right onto a road that branches out to another going to the left, on the way to Hamburg Heaven. He's never eaten in the place, but whenever he comes home from the hospital, there's always a crowd of vehicles clustered about the whitewashed building which somehow resembles a Mexican jail. That maladjusted assortment of vehicles, of a variety which he's heard his kids describe as "cool", are more often than not rust-corroded, painted with weird designs, tarnished, scraped, and missing most nonessential pieces of their exterior anatomy--but they must somehow have been able to run under their own steam to have reached this destination.

In fact, his truck is the subject of envious stares. Eat your heart out, he thinks as he eases between a converted hearse and a small van tattooed with the bumper stickers of every watering place on the eastern seaboard. The occupants glance up at him and Miriam, sitting so unnaturally high on the seats puffed up to another level by the cushions. Bairstow looks around, king of all he surveys, staring down from his perch upon the occupants of the surrounding vehicles, across at others. The boys in back wave familiarly at the crowd, content as puppies in a nest.

"Here," he says, peeling off two 10-dollars bills from his wallet and handing them through the cab's back window to the boys, "get hamburgs, will you? For your mother and me, everything on 'em including onions and pickles. You want everything on yours, don't you, Miriam?"

She smiles over at him. "Of course, Ben. It puts hair on your chest, I've heard. At least that's what you told me once in college, maybe the last time we bought hamburgs. So it should prove interesting in the very least."

How does she remember all those things, he wonders. He doesn't doubt at all that's what he said, because her mind is like a trap. She can remember conversations with people 15 years ago, people who he's long since forgotten.

They wait while the boys insinuate themselves into the mob of people cramming into the small building where hamburgs are dispensed. Bairstow hopes they won't get ptomaine or trichinosis or even typhoid in this place. He bends forward to see if he can locate the kitchen, visualizing the malevolently fierce little organisms floating in a pink sea of agar and causing the latter disease, even though he hasn't thought of it since medical school. The curse of doctors, he thinks, is that they can picture the damn bugs and visualize their primordial forms, skulking around the human race just waiting to pounce. But maybe I should get away more often, he thinks, relax and try to forget about germs for a while. When was the last time they'd gotten away, anyway?

"Miriam, would you like to take a vacation?" he asks her. "Just the two of us, I mean?"

Miriam turns her head to look at him; she, too, has been peering doubtfully at Hamburger Heaven. "Why...where do you want to go, Ben? I mean, what would we do when we got there?"

"Well..." He thinks about it. "I don't know. We could go to a warm place and go swimming."

"But that's what we do when you go to medical meetings. I swim. You don't like to swim. You sunburn."

It was true, the curse of red-haired, light-complected people. So much for that idea. "Well, we could go sightseeing. Maybe we could go to Europe."

"But you don't like airplanes. You said last time we took a transcontinental jet that you'd never go to Europe again, that those damned little seats gave you the willies, and that your spine had fused in one position. Don't you remember?"

He remembers now. He loathes sitting still, he can't bear it. Most doctors he knows are like that, they can't sit. Still, he could try. There were lots of things he could endure if he put his mind to it. "Let's think about it," he says. "You've always wanted to see Versailles and the Louvre, and I've always wanted to see St. Peter's. We shouldn't let ourselves forget that, Miriam. It's really important. Why not do some of these things we've wanted to do for so long? Don't you agree?"

Miriam looks over at Bairstow, open surprise on her face. "Are you feeling all right, Ben?"

"Perfectly."

"Why...all right. I'm game if you are. It does sound very... exciting."

"Well, remind me to think about it, and we'll make plans. Start a list, will you? There are lots of things I want to think about that I never have before."

Miriam glances at him curiously again: somehow this Bairstow isn't the same man she's known all these years, the one she's learned to cope with. This is someone different. He isn't quite like anything he's indicated he was in past years, and she's wondering how to assimilate him...as if he's a little alien around the edges. She doesn't know where he's coming from, but she's a philosophical woman. All she can do is wait and see what happens...and make that list.

The boys are back with the hamburgers, fries, and onion rings, and little plastic envelopes of condiments. For the first time all day Bairstow feels hungry--even at lunch with June he hadn't eaten well.

The boys climb back into the pickup with their paper plates, a supply of ketchup packets, and most of the fries and onions. Bairstow tucks two napkins into his shirt, suddenly realizing that he's still dressed in his office suit, and that the hamburger roll, designed to soak up juice from the patty, hasn't fully performed its function. "Damndest thing to eat," he mutters, holding the flimsy plate beneath the burger while he steers it to his mouth. "Who in hell's got a jaw that big, anyway?" Yet he takes a dogged bite from the roll.

"You asked to come, not me," says Miriam, separating the roll from the hamburg and eating them independently from each other. "You thought this would be fun."

"I know. And it is. But I just hope we don't catch something awful and end up in the emergency room. Then we can all get our pictures taken by Ebersole in his dumpy office..." So that's it. He's back with June again, thinking of her uncertain future.

Miriam puts her hand on his arm. "Ben, I'm having a good time here, with you and the boys. Do you think you could relax, please? You're driving me out of my skin. And *my* hamburger's delicious. What did you expect, filet mignon?"

Of course, she's right. All of his married life, Miriam's been solid and sensible. While he's spent his life endlessly studying, first in medical school, then in internship, finally in residency, Miriam of necessity had to develop her own skills. She was a legal secretary for a while, before Amanda was born. Since then she's managed him, Amanda, the twins, the house, her own life, and God knows what else. Bairstow suspects that he's been the worst of it. Miriam," he asks her all of a sudden, "do you love me?" Strange, in this damned truck, to be discussing the essential verities.

To his astonishment, Miriam laughs. "Do I *what*?" she asks, leaning toward him.

"Love me?" he asks again, not feeling intimidated. "I don't mean the stuff in books. Do you really *love* me--like you'd die if I went away?"

Her face is in shadow. She's put down her hamburg. "But you *don't* go away, Bairstow. I told you, you won't even go to Europe."

That's it, then: there's no answer? He'll never know for sure?

Miriam leans forward and places her hand on his arm. "I *love* you, my darling husband. I'd die if you went away. I don't know what I'd do without you. And I mean all of those things with my whole heart, you silly. Now does that make you feel better?"

He looks at Miriam, feeling her hand on his sleeve. He takes it and holds it, putting his fingers through hers, the way they used to do when they were courting. She loves him, he knows it as surely as her hand is in his. "Thank you, Miriam," he says. "I feel better. I really do."

She withdraws her hand. "Then eat your hamburg. It's not half-bad, you know."

It isn't, really, but he has sympathy for the steer, who couldn't have been treated that well to have ended up in such inelegant surroundings. He vows that it will be a while before he suggests hamburgers again, even if everyone is thoroughly enjoying himself, as they all seem to be.

The boys finish with devil dogs, a marshmallow creation, and Miriam has coffee--Bairstow thinks he's survived so far and won't tempt fate by eating anything else. Then he starts up the old truck, and they head home. Behind them, the twins are singing a school song, and snatches of the words drift in their open windows: "...good old Bunker High, eow-eow-eow, we'll slash and tear..."

"My God, what are they teaching the kids over there?" Bairstow asks. "That's the official version?"

Miriam nods, a lingering smile on her lips. "They're the Wildcats, you know. But you don't have to worry, they're last in the league."

Bairstow has almost forgotten that the boys watch high school football practice almost every day after school, hoping they'll mirculously fill in their frames sufficiently to make the team--but Bairstow's glad for once that they're skinny. He's seen too many football injuries, having helped Seligman, the orthopedist, put knees back together in surgery. He doesn't want the twins limping through life.

At home, he parks the old truck in the "carport", the remains of an old barn at the rear of the property. It *has* been a good time. Perhaps he's becoming somewhat cantankerous and unyielding in his relationships. He and Miriam don't socialize often. Medical meetings don't count; they're so superficial. He also sees patients superficially, he helps them through a crisis, then they leave until the next crisis. He's wondered sometimes what his patients are really like away from the hospital, away from the staff...away from *him*. Different. In the privacy of their own homes, they're different. So is he. Perhaps he should go along with his own family more and allow them their different-ness also. June said as much. Yes, he's been inflexible sometimes, but he's that way with himself. He wouldn't be the surgeon he is without discipline, dedication, drive. Maybe I *am* going through a midlife crisis, Bairstow thinks--Barsamian even warned the middle-aged staff members about it at a luncheon a month or so ago. Everyone had laughed and made lame jokes about their sex drives going berserk, but none of it had made much sense. Maybe Barsamian is going through a mid-life crisis of his own, Bairstow speculates, because he's divorcing his wife of ten years for a younger woman and taking on three young children besides. Maybe *he* ought to see a psychiatrist. Bairstow permits himself the hint of a smile as he trudges back from the perimeter of the property thinking of Barsamian confessing his sins to another shrink, even as he, Bairstow, used to confess his sins to Father Grogan and the Catholic church in his confessional.

Over the line he sees Herb Mathewson digging in the scrubby woods behind his garage. He doesn't feel particularly like talking to Herb, but the man suddenly turns and sees him, waves a gloved hand, and Bairstow moves to the rocky wall dividing the properties. "What are you doing?" he calls amiably to Herb. "Burying a body?"

Herb ambles over: he's a cadaverously thin man who perpetually wears a small felt hat on his head. He's always looked to Bairstow like the Jeff of Mutt and Jeff, the old comic strip Bairstow remembers from his childhood. For some reason Herb is dragging his shovel over with him. Before his retirement he'd owned a successful car dealership down by the highway. He has two grown children living in the Midwest somewhere, and Bairstow doesn't particularly like him because he considers the man to be a social climber, striving to entertain only the most prominent people.

"Trying to start a mulch pile," Mathewson says. "Edith says we've got to have a mulch pile, everyone else has one. How the hot shit does one start a mulch pile, anyway?"

Bairstow knows, but doesn't much feel like elaborating--he's feeling pooped now and wants to retreat into his house. He wants to call June, to see if Potter's returned. "You've got to collect all the grass clippings, potato peelings, everything, in one place and cover it with dirt, Herb. I've got a book about it. Do you want to borrow it?"

Mathewson shrugs. "Sure. Edith says it saves money on fertilizer. Anything to save money, I always say."

Mathewson's a stingy miser--probably he spends too much on booze for his parties with the "right" people--he wouldn't spend the money to purchase a book himself. But the guy's a neighbor after all. "I'll send one of the kids over with it, Herb," Bairstow says. "Edith's right, it does save money. And it's better by far than fertilizer. I use mulch on those peonies on the border." The peonies are a sore point between Bairstow and Mathewson: Bairstow's have bloomed as if the plants had somehow exploded into color, and Mathewson's, on the same border, appear droopy and pale in comparison.

Mathewson looks over at Bairstow as if he's finally broken Bairstow's secret code. He grasps the shovel more firmly in his hand. "Well, thanks, Bairstow. Guess I better get to work on the damn things or Edith will have my head." He appears happier to Bairstow than he's seen him in months. "Looks like Amanda's out on a toot," he says, turning away. "Don't know how they fit so many people in one car. Growing up, that girl."

Amanda's out on a date, Bairstow deciphers, probably with that Mafia chieftain and a group of his henchmen, and she's acting pretty much like a hussy. But then, Bairstow reasons, Mathewson would disapprove of the Virgin Mary without a formal gown.

Bairstow's cell phone signal goes off, and he moves away from Mathewson to answer it, walking toward the house as he goes. One of his patients has slipped and is afraid he's ruptured his wound. "Get the emergency room physician to look at it," Bairstow tells the nurse. "Who's on?"

"Dr. Gorman, sir."

"Jeez!" exclaims Bairstow. "Not Gorman." Not that damn ass, he says to himself, but he's still sorry he said what he did aloud. Gorman's already screwed up two of his cases this month and he doesn't want to give him a crack at another. "I'll be right down," he tells the nurse.

He waves to Miriam; by now she's so used to his abrupt comings and goings that she barely looks up from removing a splinter from Norman's finger. "So long, Dad," the boy yells, waving his free hand at him. "Thanks for the burgers."

Bairstow drives to the hospital: there's little traffic, he'll have no trouble. It's rush hour that does his coronaries in. Gorman has bad judgment, in Bairstow's opinion: his stitches pull out and his wounds don't heal. There's no blaming Gorman specifically because the man is properly trained and he's practiced a long time, but he has trouble entirely too much of the time, defying the percentages of wounds that ought to heal, and Bairstow doesn't trust him near his post-ops. Besides, the man who's fallen is seventy and a slow healer--Bairstow knows he'll need a little extra coddling. In addition, he's a dignified man with a sense of humor and a brain full of wonderful, odd information, a genuine charmer. He'd taught in an Ivy League school before he retired.

At the hospital, the old gentleman is already in the care of nurses, is undressed and prone on the examining table when Bairstow arrives. Bairstow greets him, then immediately begins to probe around the wound, which looks pink but shows no danger of rupturing. To make sure, Bairstow asks for the magnifying lens from one of the nurses.

"Your Boswell glasses?" the old professor asks with a smile. "What do you see through them, Dr. Bairstow? A wry world, like Dr. Johnson's?"

The assisting nurse misunderstands. "Dr. Kulick says he can see right through all our dresses," she says. "I hope it isn't true. But I always wear my black underwear just in case."

Hospital conversation is fundamental, Bairstow knows, and he enjoys it most of the time except in the operating room. He thinks his patients do, too, but he doesn't like to push it. "What *do* you see through that lens?" the old man asks, watching Bairstow's face.

"A vein that looks like a garden hose," Bairstow answers. "Magnified, your incision is like a railroad track, wandering all over the place as if I were drunk when I did it. My fingers through these Boswell spectacles resemble sausages; they get in my way. It takes a special technique to use the instrument."

The old man laughs. "Boswell would have been fascinated. He might even have thought they focused on something worth looking at, Dr. Bairstow. That's an inside joke, because Boswell asked Dr. Johnson once if a certain bridge over the Thames wasn't worth looking at, and Johnson replied that it was, but not worth going to *see*. I'm sure neither Boswell nor Johnson would have thought it was worth your coming to see my poor wound, either, and I'm sorry to get you out, Doctor, but appreciate it very much, anyway."

After the professor leaves, Bairstow closes up shop: he may be back in ten minutes or in ten hours or not at all. He calls June from the empty doctors' office: he's been waiting to call her all evening but hasn't had the opportunity. "How are you?" he asks when she answers. "Has Potter returned yet, June?"

"Not yet, Ben."

So Potter still doesn't know. He'd feared as much. "What are you doing right now?"

"Reading. I always read in the evening. And I was thinking of you, how nice you were to come over today. Why, I almost feel...beholden to you. How's that for a good old-fashioned word?"

"I've done nothing, June. I'm not sure I like the word very well. You don't owe me anything."

"I know it, Ben. That's what's so great about it. I feel your...what is it?...empathy. I told you before that I felt that in you. That's priceless, by the way, freely given and freely accepted. It comes from the heart. Have you always been this way? I mean, Jeff never says much about you. I'm sorry to say that--it's not because he doesn't admire you. He just never talks about medicine, only bicycle racing."

Unfortunately that sounds like Potter. "Maybe that's really the way we are. It's something I read--I have it here somewhere, in this damned journal--oh yes, here it is. It says that surgeons score high on tests measuring aggression, dominance, endurance, perseverance, cynicism, compulsiveness, and memory for facts and details. I find that shattering. I didn't think we were such beasts. Hold on, it gets worse. This guy says we're traditional, not very reflective, and score lowest on introspection, emotional support and humanitarianism." He laughs unhappily and shakes his head. "Maybe I should go bicycle riding, too, to escape the image. I'd give anything not to be the stereotype, but maybe I have been in the past. However, in my defense, I'd like to cite recent improvement, and the optimistic feeling I carry in my breast that maybe it will last."

June is silent for a moment. "I doubt you've ever been the stereotype, Ben. But I'd be delighted to write the author of that survey and tell him what I think of it..and of him. I could even give you a testimonial..."

Bairstow begins to feel lighter, more buoyant. "I appreciate the good words, June, but the guy might turn out to be the stereotypical survey-taker who deals only in platitudes. Have you thought of that?"

He can hear her soft chuckle. "I'd rather not. Now maybe you'll tell me what you really called for."

Bairstow closes the medical journal he'd been quoting and throws it into the wastebasket at his feet. "I want you to tell Potter promptly about your health when he returns. No maybes, ifs, or buts. I don't want Potter after my scalp, but that's not the reason. You need the moral, physical and whatever other support he can give you. I want to consult with him about it, too. It's about time he put aside that bicycle for a while to give you solace. I think he's been a little kid about long enough."

He can hear June's sharp intake of breath. "You want *me* to tell him *that?*"

"Not all of it. I'll tell him myself if I have to. I'm supposed to be insensitive, right? You have no idea how insensitive I can be if the necessity for it arises."

She's still breathing through the mouthpiece sufficiently audibly so that he can hear her. "I'll tell him, Ben. I told you I would."

"I mean now. As soon as he comes home. Give him a chance to be a man, June. He may surprise you and rise to the occasion."

Her voice sounds thoughtful. "All right, I promise. What will I do if he doesn't..."

"We'll worry about that if he doesn't."

There's another silence. "Maybe I don't give him a chance..."

"Maybe you don't. Now go to sleep. You don't have to read all night, you know. Get some rest. I'll think of you."

"And I of you."

He hangs up the phone and reaches for the coat he's thrown onto the arm of the threadbare couch. Someone ought to fix up this doctors' room, he thinks testily. It's a disgrace, an occupational hazard. I'm going to call a staff meeting to tackle it--I'll be damned if I'm going to copy Ebersole in maintaining a resident dump.

CHAPTER THIRTEEN

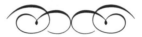

The call comes in early in the morning: the telephone beside his bed jangles, and he can feel Miriam stir. "Bairstow," he says to identify that he's awake, but his voice is heavy with sleep, and his brain is not keeping pace.

The voice of the nurse is urgent. "Dr. Bairstow, there's been an automobile accident. Can you come right down? They're here in emergency now."

By now Bairstow has started to make sense of the words; usually it doesn't take him long. "All right. What time is it, anyway?" He glances toward the lighted bedside clock, now that his eyes are beginning to focus.

"Going on three, I'm afraid."

"What's the trouble, Sandy?" He's known the woman for fifteen years, she's been the mainstay of the emergency room, and she sounds stiff and uneasy.

"We think one of the women in the accident is your daughter, sir."

Now Bairstow comes full awake, blinking to clear his sight and head. Amanda? Jesus God! "I'll be right down, Sandy. How bad is it?"

"We don't know, sir. But she's alive, if that's what you mean. Broken bones...the rest we're trying to identify. She was sitting in the back seat, luckily. The couple in the front seat are both dead."

Bairstow throws on his clothes. For a moment he bends to awaken Miriam, then decides against it: he'll straighten things out as best he can, then call her when there's something to report. For now she'd only worry...terribly.

He races through the dark. He's done it dozens, hundreds of times, but not for his own daughter. He's sometimes thought that this car could go on without him, even making right turns at red lights, to arrive of its own volition in the hospital parking lot. But tonight he's giving the driving every bit of the energy in his body, fighting the steering wheel for every last iota of control and screeching around corners. By the time he rounds the last curve, he can already see the lights in the emergency room in the next block. An ambulance is parked before the wide doors of the covered entryway. Probably it's the ambulance that brought them in. Good Christ, he thinks. He tries to keep himself under control, and finds that he can barely manage: his own shock is palpable. Maybe he'll begin to function again in a few minutes, after the pain and reality have settled in. He's seen it happen in his patients, but he can't compose himself at this minute. There are other people in the waiting room appearing tense and stricken. He hurries past them, incurring glares because for some reason he's being allowed into the inner sanctum beyond, and they have no idea that it's because he's a doctor. Sandy is waiting for him. She looks at him with sympathy and without a word leads him to the first gurney beyond the first ring of sheets hanging from metal room dividers.

There she is, flat on the gurney, her eyes barely open. Her face is a mass of bruises and cuts. Sandy or one of the other nurses has placed bandages on some of the cuts, but others are still oozing blood. Her leg has been broken, judging from the angle and the way it's propped, and she's being given pain-killing medication as well as blood. "Hi," she mutters when she recognizes Bairstow. Her voice is barely audible and plaintive, like a little girl's, and it makes Bairstow want to cry.

"Hi, Amanda. How are you doing?" He was about to add, "darling" but doesn't know how Amanda would take it. No reason to ask how it happened, only how she's faring. Bairstow will find out the details from the attending emergency room physician soon. "Are you in pain?"

She shakes her head. Her pupils are wide with the drug. "It was… awful," she whispers. "Everyone was yelling. Are the others all right?"

"I don't know," Bairstow lies. "I just got here." He can see no reason to bombard her already damaged psyche with additional shock at this juncture.

"My leg hurts," she says, feebly moving her hand as if to reach it. "It's so sore."

"It's broken," says Bairstow. "Wait, I'll find out what's going on. Back in a minute." He leaves the sheet-enclosed area to find the emergency room physician. He almost runs into the man, Jack Helmsman, just beyond the patients' area, near the desk. The man is breathless, hurrying from one room to the other, and grasps Bairstow's arm briefly in apology. "Tough, Bairstow. I'm damned sorry," he says. "But she's doing better than the others." Bairstow can see in Helmsman's hand the forms which have to be filled out when there are deaths. Bairstow has never, ever in his life, felt as bereft as at this moment. He feels himself struggling for his professionalism, hoping it will come to his aid soon. He needs anything to latch onto, as if he's adrift from every familiar mooring he's ever known.

"I'll be glad to help," he tells Helmsman. "But, for God's sake, what happened, Jack?"

Helmsman shrugs. "They've been too out-of-it to get the story straight. We've been up to our necks handling the injuries. Two died, you know that. The fourth passenger has head injuries, he may not live. We just shipped him out to the Center to the neurosurgeons."

"Dark-haired, olive skin, moustache?" Bairstow asks. He figures that if the windshield in front killed the two passengers, the man in back was with Amanda and might have been the one in the restaurant yesterday.

Helmsman turns away: he's filling out forms as he talks. "Damned if I know, Ben. Yes, come to think of it, that's the guy. Head too bruised to notice. It's in the hands of the police now, but they know who the driver was so it's pretty routine."

So her companion was that Mafia type, Bairstow thinks...but he doesn't mean it that way; in a sense Bairstow feels sorry for him, despite the fact that he undoubtedly tried to seduce Amanda and lead her down the primrose path to her own destruction. He almost got her killed, Bairstow judges--and then gets hold of himself again, because the man has almost done himself in as well.

"How's Amanda, Joe?" He himself saw on the form what part of the diagnosis is, but he wants to hear it from Helmsman's mouth.

"Broken leg, severe contusions, cuts on her face. We've called in Goldman to tidy things up, Ben. And Baringer. X-rays are in the works."

That explains what Bairstow needs to know: Goldman is the plastic surgeon who may have to repair Amanda's face. She may not look too pretty for a while. Baringer's the orthopedic surgeon who'll set the leg. Thank God if those are the only people she'll need to reunite the pieces of her body.

Time to call Miriam; at least everything's been done that can be done, and the blood's been cleaned up. He heads to the phone in the single private office in this department and closes the door. Many a time he's called members of other families to tell them the sad news, but never his own.

The telephone rings only twice. It's now 3:30. Miriam will at first think it's a call for him, that she can roll over and go back to sleep until she looks over and discovers that he's already gone. Why would they call if he's already at the hospital, she'll wonder. This will shatter what's left of her night: she won't turn back to sleep again after his message.

"Hi," says Bairstow when he hears her voice. "Sorry to wake you up."

"What's wrong, Bairstow?" Her voice is tense and urgent.

He marvels at her; in a single moment she's put together the fact that this has nothing to do with his business, that it's something else, that the vibrations between them are signaling an alarm.

"It's Amanda, Miriam. She's been in an accident, but she's pretty much all right. She's alive, a few broken..."

"I'll be right over." No histrionics, nothing. She hangs up. She'll be here, thinks Bairstow looking at his watch, in about eighteen minutes. That's his record, and she'll shatter it tonight. He returns to Amanda.

She's still awake in her groggy torpor, dully watching his face appear at her stretcher-side.

"Your mother's on her way," says Bairstow, taking her limp hand from the covers and holding it between his own. "Try to look well so you don't scare her to death, all right?" Then he hopes she knows he meant his lame joke to cheer her, that he isn't being callous. One never knows with Amanda, and he's surprised at himself that he took the chance. To his relief, she smiles wanly. He goes on. "You're going to be all right, darling." This time the endearment comes out unbidden. "They'll set your leg and put some bandages on your face. Dr. Goldman's coming over to take a look, he ought to be here soon." He notices her stir, the first agitation he's noticed, and stops. "Don't worry, Amanda, Goldman's a fine surgeon, he's our miracle worker around here. Baringer's on his way, too. Try to rest until they come."

Miriam arrives in seventeen minutes flat, which Bairstow finds unbelievable because she doesn't leave her clothes in a neat pile on the hall chair as he does in anticipation of these frantic rushes. Miriam is fully dressed, although she's without her color and lipstick.

"How'd it happen?" she asks, grasping Bairstow's arm. "Where is she?"

Bairstow leads her into the emergency room, explaining as he goes. "Crashed into a cement road divider," he says. "Two died, the other's in serious shape. She's groggy but awake."

Miriam enters the area while Bairstow pushes back the hanging drapes. She immediately bends to kiss Amanda's forehead, then collapses onto the chair beside her daughter's bed, stretching her arm protectively across her body. "Darling..." she murmurs. "Oh, darling..."

Amanda slowly opens her eyes. "Hi," she says in a thin voice, as she had with Bairstow. "You...came."

Miriam flashes a look at Bairstow. "You think I wouldn't?" Her hand is smoothing Amanda's bedclothes, as if soothing her as well. "Besides, there wasn't a thing on the Late, Late Show anyway."

Crazy humor runs in our family, thinks Bairstow. Even when Amanda is lying here in desperate condition, we can't help it. Anyone listening would think we're crazy. But Amanda smiles...and *that*, thinks Bairstow, was Miriam's intent in the first place.

Just then they hear Baringer's booming voice--he's coming to set Amanda's leg. Baringer lives across town, in a rural area where his wife raises sheep, using the wool for weaving. It always takes him half the night to get to the hospital. Bairstow can never understand how the man puts up with his commuting distance, but that's Baringer's business, not his. At least he's arrived to assist his child.

Bairstow knows Baringer pretty well: they're always thrown together for one reason or another, not the least of which is that their names follow in the alphabet. Their lockers in the dressing room abut. Baringer likes to tell loud, booming jokes, leaving Bairstow to wonder why he likes the man, but he does.

"Well, what have we got here?" asks Baringer, standing beside the gurney after he's said hello to Miriam and raised his hand to Bairstow. "You've been trying to kick the hell out of a cement barricade, young lady? Tell you the truth, you won't win. Now let's take a look at that leg and see where we go from here."

The minute Baringer handles Amanda's numbed leg, Bairstow knows it's going to be no simple job: her foot moves awkwardly out of position. It's obvious that both major bones have been broken, and from the way Miriam gives a little start and turns pale, he knows that she realizes it, too. It will be months before Amanda walks freely again, and she may have to spend much of that time in traction.

Baringer looks over at Bairstow and nods. "Might as well do it now," he says, rubbing his chin thoughtfully. "Tomorrow's a shitter of a day, surgery all morning and most of the way through the afternoon." He sticks his head through the wall of sheets and calls for Sandy, then begins to explain his plan of attack to Bairstow, talking constantly and gesturing. "Sooner we put that pin in, the sooner she's gonna be out dancing the fandango, Ben. Besides, she's medicated now and half out of it so's we won't have to add too much to the brew, if you see what I mean."

Bairstow wonders what patients must think of Baringer. Lots of good things, he realizes, because the man's waiting room is always filled to the rafters with men, women, kids and old ladies. Yet if his wild, usually off-color, stories in the operating room and the high profile he likes to maintain combine to offend Bairstow's upbringing, for some odd reason they entertain him at the same time. He's never met anyone quite like Baringer, but he wouldn't want the man around for very long at a stretch. When Baringer turns to him and asks, "If you'd assist, I'd be damned grateful, Ben," Bairstow understands full well that Baringer is hard up because there are no other surgeons around at this time of night, though one could be summoned. Amanda's his own daughter, and one thinks twice about treating one's own kin, but it's only assisting, after all, which amounts to nothing more than prepping the involved limb, holding retractors, and following Baringer's lead.

When Bairstow nods in acquiescence, Baringer, still carrying on at the top of his lungs, summons his team, dispatching Sandy to make some of the calls, and departing to make arrangements. Bairstow and Miriam watch over Amanda: she's teetering on the brink of sleep. In a minute Ferraro or his assistant will arrive to begin anesthesia, and within a half-hour when the room is ready they'll get under way. The rest of this night is going to be a long one.

Miriam looks at her watch: Bairstow has been with Amanda in the operating room for three hours and fifteen minutes now. She knows it won't take much longer but she feels restless. Bairstow has arranged for her to sit in the doctors' lounge, which is empty, and she waits there alone wishing she'd chosen instead to sit outside in the public waiting room so she could observe other people coming and going. But, she thinks, it's nice to sit here in the semi-dark and let my thoughts float, which I couldn't do if I had others around. She feels that whatever gods there are must have all smiled on Amanda at the same time to have allowed her to survive this terrible ordeal. Miriam has been murmuring a prayer, a supplication from deep in her religious past, since that devastating moment when Bairstow first called her. She can't even remember the prayer or where she heard it: Lord God, she'd repeated over and over, as if her own voice were on a recording, let her be alive, Lord God let her stay alive. Even though Bairstow had said she'd survive, Miriam had been afraid he'd been trying to soften the blow and she wouldn't ultimately make it. She feels as if they all must have done something right to have willed Amanda through this calamity relatively unscathed, but for the life of her she can't think what she and Bairstow might have done right to deserve this blessing, that their daughter will live when others have died. But she doesn't want to question too much, either, for fear her guardian angel might remember that she's occasionally sinned. All she wants to do right now is dwell in the miraculous knowledge that her daughter really is alive, however battered her body.

It astonishes Miriam that when the chips are down she so readily invoked the name of the deity, for she's thought that she'd let religion slip a long while ago, somewhere in the prehistoric past of her adolescence. Distantly she can remember going to church every Sunday, and to the church school, too. Unlike Bairstow, she's still gone to church occasionally, and here it is, her faith showing itself in this hard time of Amanda's sad night. She's heard that, during agonizing convolutions of the spirit, religion sometimes emerges again--and that's the way it seems to be happening with her, drawing on roots from her youth. She wonders what the parents of the two dead children are going through; she can hardly bear to think of it, because her own pain is so intense...and her child is actually alive! She's said more than once that she thought the worst thing in life must be to lose a child, and tonight she's thought she might have to face it, but thank God, thank God, she didn't!

She can't stay indefinitely: she'd awakened the twins before she left and told them what little she knew of Amanda's condition before she placed them under their own recognizance. She'd done it before: after all, they are twelve. *They* consider themselves at twelve to be virtually adult, but at least they're sufficiently capable of keeping themselves out of trouble for a few hours. The twins will be anxious to hear what's happening with their sister, too, although they know that she's survived.

She looks across the room toward the door where Bairstow disappeared so long ago. Poor Amanda is going to have metal pins through her leg temporarily, the kind that penetrate skin, bone and muscle to make one resemble a shish kebab. There'll be pain, but that's all right, too, Amanda can stand the pain. It's a hard lesson, a terribly hard, indecently hard lesson, though. Other children belonging to close friends have died in the same tragic way. Some were stoned on drugs, they'd never known what hit them--or who they'd hit with their vehicles. The son of an internist once swallowed a handful of pills for kicks, then had lain down in the road after becoming convinced that cars would float over him--at least that's what he'd told his companions, equally stoned, before he died. The first car hadn't floated, it had run over him in the dark instead. The boy was only 14.

But Amanda is not a child any longer; she's an adult, a responsible human. She lives at home as a child only occasionally now; even then her room seems to the family like an armed camp, where she can keep them all away. It's a fortress for pain, like a boil on the epidermis of their family life, but at least Amanda is alive, alive, alive nearby, not at a distant hospital somewhere miles away. And thank God she's not in the bowels of this hospital where they've taken the other two, to be dispatched to a funeral home. She'd overheard the nurses talking matter-of-factly about the two who didn't survive when they thought everyone was out of earshot. Well, she'll try to manage this: maybe she has more self-control than some because she's dealt with life and death through Bairstow for years now, but she knows very well that she couldn't handle herself if it had been one of her children who had died.

Yes, Amanda must become an adult. Bairstow had said it and he was right. Her adolescence is over; this accident will almost guarantee it. What a pity to lose your youth this way. But, thinks Miriam, she and Bairstow were married at Amanda's age, but younger marriages were more in fashion then. They'd simply fallen in love and couldn't stand being apart, so they'd married, just like that. They'd had a good life together, a good marriage, and she didn't regret it at all. He'd been faithful—probably; she had been, without question. She actually didn't care whether Bairstow had been faithful or not, nurses were after him all the time. She had merely to place her leg against his at night, and he was there, wanting her. If he'd ever cared for anyone else, he'd kept it to himself, and for that she was grateful. She had him, body and soul, and that's all she wished for. It was all of him, really.

But she knows that Bairstow is somehow aware of something about this man who'd been injured with Amanda: there'd been that ripe hesitancy when Bairstow first heard of him. She'd known full well that Bairstow hadn't approved of the man, and that his disapproval had nothing to do with squeamishness about his daughter's dating (many men felt challenged when their daughters began to date, but Bairstow wasn't one of them). Maybe he's met the man elsewhere, Miriam thinks, but where? Perhaps he'd treated him for something--my God, could it be gonorrhea? *That* would upset Bairstow no end, infuriate him, drive him wild. She could ask him right out if he knows this Mario, but he might have to violate a medical confidence to answer, and besides, what difference does it make, anyway? Nor does it matter if they'd been drinking, or high on drugs, as long as they're alive. Amanda is alive, her darling daughter, her wonderful child. What does it matter that she's been difficult, as long as she's alive?

She suddenly realizes that the probation officer for Amanda's shoplifting conviction will have to be notified of her inability to appear before him because she's confined to the hospital. "I'm glad of that, at least," Miriam murmurs aloud, thinking that her daughter won't have to make that shameful trip to the courthouse this once, although undoubtedly the treks do Amanda good, and maybe someday will even succeed in making her privately repentant, although Mirium doubts very much that she will live to see the day.

An hour or so later Miriam hears the sound of voices in the hall: she's fallen asleep in the peaceful dark of the room. When the door pushes open, there's Bairstow, looking weary, and Baringer followed by Goldman. So they've fixed her face and her leg at the same time. She wonders about Amanda's spirit: who will fix that? But then she thinks, no need to worry about that, Amanda will come out all right...at least she's young, and the young can get through anything.

Bairstow is holding the round hat from his scrub suit in his hand. "She's out of the O.R.," he says, almost as if Miriam had asked the question.

"We can talk to her, Ben?"

He shakes his head wearily. "She'll be groggy until morning. The X-rays show broken ribs, so Baringer set those, too. It took a while. Don't worry, Mimi. She'll be all right. Let's go home. It's been one hell of a night."

She knows moments are precious and rare when he calls her Mimi. Miriam turns to look at her husband again: he's reaching for their coats, hers and his. He means it, he's going home, they're going home together, right now, even if Amanda has to stay.

He turns at her hesitation. "She'll be in recovery the rest of the night, Miriam. Don't worry, they'll look after her. Do you realize that it's after six and I'm still on call? Except that Helmsman said he'd cover because he'll be here anyway...and Kulick volunteered, too. Nice of them. I feel a little as if a truck ran over me."

They walk silently through the hospital, past the mazes of dead ends and cul-de-sacs where Miriam always gets lost, in the inner recesses of the hospital among the laboratories, offices and examining rooms. Miriam suddenly feels surprisingly awake, she could almost sing for some ridiculous reason. The stars outside are bright as polished gems. They decide to drive a single car home; she can pick up hers tomorrow. When she offers to drive the Lexus home, Bairstow agrees without hesitation; it's rare when he'll relinquish the wheel of the Lexus even to her, but tonight is novel in every way.

She drives carefully onto the highway, taking the first exit, then steps on the accelerator and lets the car surge into the fast lane. She turns on the radio, allowing the music from an all-night FM station to flow from the speakers, soothing and restful.

A few miles into the drive, she hears an odd, buzzing sound. She looks quickly around: she isn't familiar with Bairstow's car, and thinks that there's a buzzer warning her that something imminent will occur if she isn't on guard to prevent it. But she can't find a thing wrong--no light on the dashboard, nothing.

In another moment, after the sound comes to her ears again, she realizes what it is, and a smile comes to her lips: beside her, Bairstow is sound asleep, snoring. His head is thrown back, he's loosened his collar, unbuttoned his shirt, and he's in another world. She centers her attention on the road once more, and keeps pushing forward. Her brief urge to sing has long since fled, and she feels exhausted, too. Bairstow was right: it *has* been a hell of a night. She never wants to see another like it.

CHAPTER FOURTEEN

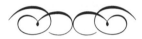

In the morning, Bairstow returns to the hospital at 7:00 a.m. both to see Amanda and to look in on a woman with post-operative cancer who is spiking a fever. First, from the hospital, he calls June to tell her what's happened. He knows that her CT scan is scheduled for tomorrow, that Potter has yet to arrive, and that she will be home.

"Oh, you poor man," June exclaims after he hears of Amanda's plight. "You must feel just dreadful."

"She could be dead or maimed, June. It could have been infinitely worse."

"I know, Ben. But how do *you* feel?"

"Tired. We were up all night."

"You're back at the hospital?"

"Unfortunately, yes."

"But why are you up so early?"

Bairstow thinks about it a minute. "Tell you the truth, I honestly don't know. My patient could have waited. And Amanda is sleeping. But I couldn't stay in bed. I feel...tense. Lord, I never felt so tense."

"Well, you have a right, you know. If you didn't, I'd wonder."

Back in the confines of the doctors' waiting room, Bairstow rubs the back of his neck. His shoulders ache. "I'm coming over," he says on a sudden resolve. "Can you stand a morning visitor?"

"Always. Have you had breakfast?"

Bairstow considers her question. "I doubt it. Somehow the day and night got mixed."

"Then I'll have something ready."

"Thanks. About an hour? First I've got to make rounds...and visit Amanda."

Amanda's room is darkened and she appears asleep. There's no one in the bed next to hers: the admission people, bless them, have managed to find her a single room, at least for now. Her leg is suspended in the air, in traction. It looks God-awfully uncomfortable, and Bairstow considers that he's lucky he never had to go through such a miserable process. Amanda's long, auburn hair is fanned out on the pillow beside her, and Bairstow is struck again by how much in repose her features looks like Miriam's.

Just as he's about to retreat, she stirs. "Hi," she murmurs in a small voice.

Bairstow enters the room fully this time. "I didn't know you were awake, Amanda. Do you feel like company?"

She nods her head slightly--and Bairstow understands without asking that it isn't from unwillingness to have him there, but that she's incredibly stiff. Every muscle, joint, and ligament in her body must ache, not counting the leg. He walks over to the bed, pulls up the small bedside chair, and straddles it. "Hi," he says, "Fancy meeting you here." Then he shakes his head and smiles. "Sorry, it wasn't funny the first time I heard it, either."

"You don't have to be funny."

All the women in Bairstow's life like to tell him the things he doesn't have to be: June, that he doesn't have to be responsible for so many others; Miriam, that he doesn't have to be available for her to lean on; now Amanda, who says that he doesn't have to be funny. This time it amuses him. "I'm not trying to be funny, I'm just trying not to be sad," he answers. "I feel sad today for many reasons, not the least of which is seeing you in that rig. Maybe when I fully wake up, I'll feel better." Actually, he *has* woken up now, and he still feels grim.

"But I don't feel so bad," Amanda answers from the bed, her voice almost wistful. "Isn't that crazy? I might have woken up dead. It was so awful."

No one has related to him just how awful it really was, and although these things rarely make him flinch, involved as he has been so intimately with broken bodies all of his professional life, he doesn't know if he can face it where his daughter is concerned. Yet maybe it will benefit Amanda to talk about it.

"The guy driving was a friend of Mario's," Amanda explains, elaborating as she goes and moving her hands feebly about in the air. "I didn't like him at all--he was stoned when he arrived. Mario tried to keep him from driving. We didn't know just how bad he was for a while. By then he was already behind the wheel." She stops, exhausted.

Bairstow knows from sad experience that initially it's hard to discern when a man is stoned from an overdose of drugs. There's no smell, as from alcohol, and usually one doesn't get close enough to observe the dilated pupils of his eyes. One of his colleagues had been required to take over from a drug-impaired physician in the operating room--even his assistant hadn't noticed the symptoms until the man's hands began to shake. Luckily, the physician has now been rehabilitated in a clinic, but another addicted doctor Bairstow heard about is a skid-row bum, having lost his grip on himself and his profession.

"Finally, Mario got mad," Amanda is continuing. "He insisted that his friend pull over. Instead, the guy floored the accelerator. We hit a bridge abutment and a cement post. At least that's what I heard one of the policemen say when I came to. Before that, I remember lights and loud noises. People were crying and yelling."

It must have been terrible, Bairstow is thinking, a nightmare for Amanda to live through. He still can't imagine how she survived, but she must have had fate on her side last night. He is eternally thankful for whatever gods saw fit to intervene on her behalf.

"Would you call up to see how Mario is doing?" Amanda asks him, her eyes turned up to his face. Her voice seems tremulous now, almost apologetic when she remembers under what unfortunate circumstances her father first encountered her friend. Bairstow can also hear the sound of fatigue in his daughter's voice as well, and doesn't know which holds precedence, apology or exhaustion, but it's a tone he's never heard before.

He slowly stands up and pats her arm. "Of course I'll call if you wish. Get some rest, I'll come in later. Your mother will be here, too, after she's had a chance to sleep."

She reaches her hand feebly to touch his, yet there's a hint of humor in her voice. "I suppose them's doctor's orders."

"You can bet your sweet bippy they are," he answers.

Before he leaves the hospital, Bairstow asks the nurses where they've taken Mario: Helsman's trying to get a little sleep and Baringer has long since gone home. The nurses consult the record, which is still on the floor and hasn't been sent on to the record room. "To Dr. James Plotkin at the Center, by ambulance," the accident room nurse reads from the chart. "They haven't reported anything else about him."

Bairstow finds Plotkin's number in the phone directory and places the call to the physician. A nurse answers at the Center, and informs Bairstow in a testy voice that Dr. Plotkin has gone to bed, that he'd spent a very hard night. "Tell me about it," Bairstow mutters aloud, feeling his own pulse hammering in his temple, and almost adding that it wasn't Plotkin's daughter who was injured. Of course, Bairstow has to concede that Plotkin has done his work for the night and has legitimately earned a few hours in the sack. Besides, Bairstow has heard good things about Plotkin and respects the precise nature of the art which neurosurgeons practice and the compulsive nitpicking of their technique. It drives Bairstow right up a wall on the few times he's been asked to assist in minor cases, yet such persnickety proceedings often achieve miraculous results from the long, arduous hours in the operating room. He hopes that Plotkin has been able to exert his considerable skills on the brain of Amanda's friend, Mario.

Yet, as Bairstow is about to hang up and depart, the nurse calls his name and indicates that they're holding an incoming call at the emergency desk. It's Plotkin's assistant, sounding tired to Bairstow's ear. Obviously, they've had a night of it over there, too.

"Thanks for calling back," Bairstow says into the phone. "We sent over a young man named Mario something-or-other, who'd been in an automobile accident. Sorry, I don't know his last name. Can you tell me what his prognosis is?"

"Guarded," the physician replies. "Very guarded. We won't know for a few days, Dr. Bairstow, if he survives that long. We spent most of the night pulling out bone fragments from his brain."

He'll probably die, Bairstow thinks, listening to the careful language of the neurosurgeon, as meticulously chosen as is his own wording when the outcome of a case is far from certain. "Guarded" is Bairstow's own term when one has made a last-ditch effort and can't forsee the outcome.

Another blow for Amanda. Not that he was enthralled with her companion; he wishes the man well but has no desire to lay every bit of sad news at her door at once.

One last call, to Miriam: he'd promised to call. She answers the phone immediately, even though it's barely dawn and ordinarily she would not have stirred by now, but this is a night like no other they've known in their lives.

"She's all right," he says quietly into the phone. "She's barely awake, Miriam. Stay in bed, there's nothing that needs doing right now. Try to get some rest yourself."

Silence for a moment: he knows from long experience that she's switching the phone from one ear to the other. "All right, Ben, I will. Thank you."

"Amanda will be awake and want to see you later in the morning. When the night's worn thin."

That's such a strange expression--"when the night's worn thin"-- almost poetic, and he can't imagine where he heard it. Well, he thinks, that's what night does, as if it's a curtain, it wears thin and then the light peaks through.

"I will, Ben. You'll be back later?"

"In a little while, yes."

The morning light is glowing in the sky as he leaves the hospital, but his spirits still feel heavy: behind him is Amanda, in that bed. He's never left behind a member of his family in a hospital bed before, except for Miriam when Amanda and the twins were born, and even then he'd spent most of his time at the hospital with her. Now he can feel the aftereffects of Amanda's accident, settling like a shock wave through his body. He may have had his differences with Amanda, but he's never realized the depth of his affection for her until now. Even at this minute he senses that not all of his suppressed feelings have boiled to the surface. He finds it terrifying even to contemplate the depth of the grief he'd have to manage if her fate had been the same as the other passengers of that car. Now Bairstow can feel his body quaking, so much that he has to drive the car with conscious control, taking it to the far right lane on the highway and clamping both hands on the glove-leather steering wheel for steadiness. He's glad that June doesn't live at a greater distance, because he doesn't think he's capable of driving much farther than her house at this moment.

When he arrives in her neighborhood, the morning sun has disappeared under a cloud bank and the day is turning rainy and overcast, which does little to lighten his mood. Yet he *can* feel a buoyancy overtaking him just knowing that he will be having breakfast with June, the thought of which has been sustaining him in some vital way since he spoke with her. He parks his car in her driveway, and when he rings the bell, he realizes that she's been waiting for him; within an eyeblink she's opened the door and ushered him inside. She's wearing a large white apron which wraps around her slim frame as if it's enclosing a mummy. She looks at his face and doesn't say a word, but takes his coat first, hanging it in the closet, then pushes open the door and ushers him into the kitchen, from which a myriad of aromatic smells are emerging. "Come inside," she says, "and we'll see what we can do to make you feel better." She's been baking bread, he can see the dough on the breadboard. "Sit down," she says, "you can watch. It seems to be my good luck to have you as the patron saint of my kitchen, Ben, watching over my meager culinary efforts."

He looks at her and realizes that from the moment he'd consented to come to breakfast, she's been in gear, organizing it for him. In the breakfast area beyond the kitchen, behind the glass wall into her garden, a table is set for two, with blue china and bright flowered napkins. Everything shines, as if it were in a greenhouse, as if this were not the dull day it had turned out to be.

"You've gone to a lot of trouble, June," Bairstow says. "I didn't want you to."

"I haven't, Ben. But it looks as if you could stand a little pampering." She indicates the kitchen bar. "It's your seat, remember? Would you like a mimosa--to start the day with a little artificial sunshine?"

With relief, Bairstow slides into one of the comfortably wide swivel chairs. He leans across the bar, toward her. "Tell you the truth, June, I never thought I'd be suffering the bends like this. We almost lost Amanda. I'm afraid, at this moment, I'm a shaking wreck of a man. You're nice to take me off the street and attempt to rehabilitate me."

She glances quickly over at him. "It doesn't have anything to do with 'nice', Ben, so please stop. I don't have to look very carefully at you across this room to see how you're suffering." She slides the drink before him. "If you'll drink this, you'll feel a lot better."

It's true, he thinks, I can now stop feeling like a remnant of quivering, collapsed humanity. I *treat* people like me: I say, "Here, my friend, what you need is a sedative, so take it easy, go on a vacation or put your feet up for a while, and try to relax." He'll try to put that advice to use on himself…somehow.

June stands before him, watching. "You suddenly look better. Don't tell me you practice mind control?"

"I wish I did. There are times when I could use it."

She smiles at him across the counter, kneading the bread as she speaks. "I didn't mean to make light of what you're going through, Ben. It must be pure hell."

"I didn't take it that way."

"By the way, how's Amanda doing?"

"Battered body, subdued soul. Going to spend a few of what should be the best days of her life in traction."

"You're serious? I didn't realize…" She stops and studies his face.

"Oh, I don't mean in terms of time. I mean in terms of anguish. They'll just seem like very long months in her young life. She'll never forget them, I'm afraid."

"You think they'll cause her irreparable damage?"

The mimosa is going down easily and, as June had predicted, it's making Bairstow's spirits rise. "Maybe they'll be the best months of her life, who knows? Maybe she'll learn a little humility, and that will save her life, too. I've known people without it, but they have a harder time than most. At least in my experience."

"It sounds reasonable."

"Well, I've thought about giving her space, as you put it, and you were right about that, too. We've still considered her our young daughter, but I've forgotten she's almost grown-up. We've been controlling, suburban parents, and I've been the worst of it. How does one learn to let the traces go, anyway? It doesn't come easily to me for some reason, I wish I knew why. I think I've been the difficult one for Amanda; it isn't Miriam she resents. And all of a sudden I don't blame her. But now her hostility has ceased because she's suffering. At least she knows that I'm trying to help her as best I can."

"I'm sure she knows that. She hasn't received help from you before?"

He shakes his head. "Not like this. Right now she has no choice, it's not as if she could run away." He looks across at her. "Do you realize how many kids born to parents who love them take off, never to return again?"

"Quite a few, I'm certain. But I've sometimes wondered...how the parents have really been. Well, I know that Amanda loves you, Ben. I could tell even at the restaurant." She reaches over and places a plate of eggs, bacon and coffeecake before him, then sets one beside him for herself. "Forget the fancy table, Ben, let's sit right here. You still look like you're in trauma." She walks to the table set in the glass alcove and returns with a single candlestick, which she lights with a thick kitchen match. "There. Not romantic, strictly utilitarian. I'll pour you another mimosa to celebrate; then I'll rub your back. You look bent over, like an old man, as if you were carrying a weight."

Bairstow straightens his shoulders. "That's the way it seems. Did you make this coffeecake this morning?"

"With my own hands. I hope you're impressed. Besides, Jeff is coming back tonight, and it's his favorite." She watches him eat, picking at her own food.

"How did his bicycle meet go? Winningly, I trust."

"He's one of the best racers in the entire New England area."

Bairstow places his fork on the plate before him. "Isn't he a little old to be trying that hard to bring home a medal? He's past the prime age for bicyclists, I presume, and he leaves you here..."

June throws her head back and laughs. "Don't try to tell *him* that. Jeff invites me but I don't want to go to bicycle meets, they make me dizzy, all that going round and round the track. Besides, I can never tell who's in the lead. Everyone's always lapping everyone else. And they have some terrible crashes--I'm always afraid one of them will be Jeff. Of course I want him home but that's not to be, so I'll have to manage...everything...myself."

"But Potter's not such a fanatic about his surgery, so why is he so balmy about bicycle racing?"

June thinks about it a moment. "I don't know, I really don't. I think it means lost youth to him. Some men go crazy, you know, when they feel 'time's winged chariot'. How about you? It doesn't bug you?"

Bairstow remembers the times at the gym when he'd worked out, lifting weights on Saturday afternoons, taking his frustration out on the punching bag. "At one time I was like that," he acknowledges. "I still work out but it's less feverish."

June glances at him, her eyes smiling, her fingers laced under her chin. "Then maybe there's hope for Jeff. Do you want me to rub your back, or do you want to stay hunched over that way?"

Bairstow straightens when he feels June's fingers moving about his back muscles. Her hands curve about his ribs and over the broad scapula, producing heat and friction against the aches he's been almost unconscious of in his weary muscles. "Oh, my God," he moans, feeling the relief. "You're sure you weren't a physical therapist in another life?"

He can hear her laughter as she works across his back. "I'm getting pretty good at it. Jeff gets knotted, too, from his riding. Painting is my one escape. Would you care to see my oils, by the way?"

He's been wanting to see her work since he met her. The walls of this room are entirely bare, except for a portrait over the fireplace, where the central figure is dressed in a bright tunic, wears a rakish blue hat, and is bent over some sort of machine in his hand. A younger Jeff, he wonders, ready for a race, working on equipment? A child? Her inventor father as a young man?

She leads him to a room beyond the kitchen, then through a small foyer; they seem to be skirting a garden which borders on the kitchen dining area. She has to unlock a door. When she shoves it open, she first crosses the room to part curtains, then touches the light switch. Instantly the room is bathed in light--it's as simple as a monk's cell, holding only a studio couch, chair, an easel, and stacks of canvases. Several hang on the walls: vivid oils depicting stylized flowers beside curved bentwood furniture grouped around tables draped in vivid fabrics. Brown plump native women sit or lean against the chairs, their breasts full and sensual. Some are dressed in bright, flowered fabrics vibrating with greens and fuchsias and deep blues and gleaming golds. They overpower this space, and Bairstow has a feeling of teeming emotion beyond these walls, of pulsing music from other worlds revealed through the canvasses as if they were windows into an exotic universe. He can't understand why he hasn't seen June's work in museums long ago, or why she doesn't at least exhibit locally.

"Brilliant," Bairstow mutters, moving from one to the other, feeling almost an assault from each. "Do you see life this way?"

She tilts her chin up, a gesture he's become used to when she's in thought. "It's the way I wish life could be. When I was a child, I painted in water colors, the brighter the better. Now I'm more comfortable with oils. Like Van Gogh, I once used oils by the pailful...but you can see, in these, that I'm more meticulous about the application: they run with color, I know that, but I use little excess paint. I guess I've refined the process. Sometimes my canvasses give people headaches."

Bairstow can understand: the intensity of the colors seem to find a focus and bore into one's consciousness. He can't think what walls would hold these large oils without making the room drab in contrast. Yet, in the right room, they would bring it to life, a large room...

"I'd love to buy one," says Bairstow, suddenly resolved. "Especially that one, with the blue bentwood chairs and the lawn beyond. Would you consider selling it to me? I know, perhaps your price is more than I can afford, and you probably don't want to part with it, but it would absolutely *inspire* my living room."

June turns to look at him, her hand resting on the frame of her easel. "You can't be serious, Ben. You'd really like one? Why, I'd gladly give it to you."

He feels shocked by her answer. "Give it to me? Then I couldn't possibly accept it. Why, these must take you weeks, even months to finish. How did you learn to paint so well? Are you self-taught, or have you taken lessons?" Bairstow inspects the canvas again, studying the brush strokes more closely.

"Jeff never told you? I have a degree in fine arts, but I educated myself long before that. I taught once, in graduate school. I mean it,

Ben, if you're serious, I'd love you to have that painting. You can take it now. No, don't look so surprised, I can't think of anyone I'd rather have a sample of my work. I'll wrap it up for you if you'd like."

"June, I simply can't..."

"Listen, Ben, merely thinking of you looking at it delights me. You know, I'd rather have a friend own my painting than exhibit to a room of cold observers and critics. My paintings are a little like my children--I want them cared for with love and tenderness."

It's almost more than Bairstow can tolerate at that moment, the offer of such a gift. He can't find words to respond. Instead, he reaches for her hand and holds it immobilized between his. "But, you see, June, it wouldn't be appropriate, it's far too generous..."

June leans against his shoulder. "I don't know how you arrived here in my life, Ben, but I'm so glad you did. It means so much to me. I almost regret the lost time, do you know that, when Jeff was operating with you all those weeks and months and I'd never even met you. Now I have, and it makes all the difference. I mean it wholeheartedly; I want you to have the painting."

Bairstow stirs, still holding her hand. Besides gratitude, he feels overwhelming tenderness for this brief interlude from his worries over Amanda which have left him shaken and depressed. He feels infinitely better simply being with her in this quiet room, a small oasis in his present chaos. And, yes, the regret had come to him as well.

Without a word, June steps out of her shoes, then her skirt. "Listen, my dear," she says, "welcome to my world. I care about you; that must be obvious by now. Welcome, oh welcome..." She pulls back the cover on the studio couch, removing the bolsters against the back, then turns to remove Bairstow's shirt; he's already shrugged off his coat. "But you've been in my world a good while now, and I've wanted you, Ben. I hope it hasn't been too obvious. But I've cared about you so, my dear..."

She pulls him down to her on the couch, and they are together, Bairstow's face against hers, their bodies touching. Bairstow can feel his body shedding its cares, focused only on June beside him. He holds off his own urgency, cupping her small breasts and kissing the nipples, fondling the fine skin about her ears and down the line of her neck. "You are so beautiful, June, so frail..." he murmurs. "A lovely...young woman. Thank God for you now."

She moves her hands down over the lean muscles of his chest onto the skin of his belly, feeling the firmness of his erection. "And for you, Ben. You are a marvelous man...and to think we are together. It's a happy thing, almost beyond belief, that I'm here with you."

It is a time unlike any other that Bairstow can remember, except when he and Mirium were first married, when their lovemaking was a kind of ecstasy, before the children and the cares of founding a home, before the draining energies of his practice. Once there had been a nurse who found her way into his bed one night when he was on duty. A brief interlude and an unexpected one--yet that, too, was far from this.

"Ben," June murmurs in his arms after the intensity of their ardor mounts, "my dear." When they climax together, June clings to him, holding him to her, her arms held tight about him. Afterward, she luxuriates in the warmth from his body and he from hers. "You are so... wonderful," she whispers again. "My dear Ben."

He cradles June in his arms, knowing he must leave soon, that this interlude must end. "Thank you for this time," he says. "For me it's almost magical...a stolen, precious hour. Life-giving, today, for me at least."

"I hope it's not the last, my dear."

"Whatever it is, I'll remember it always," Bairstow says.

"And I," she adds. "I'll hold it in my heart as long as I live."

He leaves feeling less depressed, and for the time being, elevated above care. The rain has even magically stopped as he makes his way back to the hospital.

CHAPTER FIFTEEN

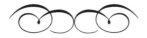

He's right, Miriam is with Amanda. He spots her car in the parking lot. In fact, he finds her sitting beside Amanda, her hand on the bed sheet. It strikes Bairstow that it's been a long while since Amanda let either of them get that close to her, but she doesn't have much choice right now. He sits down on the other side of the bed, then realizes that Amanda would have to turn both ways to see them separately, so he carries the chair around to place it next to Miriam. Miriam smiles—she's glad to see him, and he has a momentary pang having spent time with June, but he's somehow pulled through his own crisis and feels infinitely better. "How long have you been here?" he asks Miriam.

"Not long, Bairstow. Amanda was asleep when I arrived. I'm afraid I woke her up."

"No, you didn't," whispers Amanda from the bed. "I was dozing. The nurse gave me something for pain. Besides, I kept wanting to put my leg down and I started yelling at it when it wouldn't go."

The plaintive sound of Amanda's remark brings a smile to Bairstow's lips: of course she'd want to put her leg down. Who wouldn't? But it's funny, just the same. Miriam has her hand over her mouth; even Amanda is laughing, a small, apologetic laugh. It seems to Bairstow that he hasn't heard her laugh in months, maybe in years. Where had her capacity for mirth gone? Where had she lost it? But there it is, miraculously reclaimed from the verge of extinction, at Amanda's darkest hour. Bairstow has frequently seen adversity bring out peculiar results in a patient: one cantankerous old woman who threw her food dishes at the nurses left her money to the hospital, and an old man on his deathbed called in the son he'd refused to talk to for years to beg his forgiveness. Anything was possible, even Amanda laughing.

"Baringer says he'll let you out of here in a week, or perhaps even less," Bairstow tells Amanda and Miriam. "I saw him downstairs. He says some of the gross swelling has come down already. That's damned good news."

He can see Amanda assimilating that information as she touches the bandages Goldman has placed over her cheeks to unite the torn tissue. "Have you heard anythng about...Mario?" she asks.

Miriam's eyes speed to Bairstow's face. "His condition is guarded," says Bairstow. "That means that he's withstood surgery to remove bone fragments from his brain. Beyond that they don't know a thing."

Amanda's eyelids flutter, and he knows that she's alarmed but doesn't want to pry farther. But from the corner of his eye he can see Miriam staring at the floor, because she's heard the words often enough to understand that they contain little optimism and indicate a very long recuperation at best.

"Well, I don't want to tire you," Miriam says, looking again at Amanda. "You must be exhausted, my darling." She places her hand once again on Amanda's sheet. "Try to rest."

"With this thing in the air?" Amanda asks, looking up at her leg. "You must be joking."

Mirium smiles and leans to kiss her daughter. "Until later. I'll come this afternoon if you feel like it."

"Of course, Mum. I'd like it." Amanda's eyes appear enormous in the white bed, against the bandages.

Mum? Bairstow hasn't heard the word on his daughter's lips since she was four. Something has assuredly changed: temporarily she's reverted to a childlike grace. Bairstow, too, leans over her bed to kiss her forehead. His daughter's flesh is so smooth, so unlined as to be almost childlike--but she's not a child any longer, as June so forcefully pointed out. "I'll be back, too, Amanda. First I've got to get some sleep."

Miriam slips her arm through his as they walk down the hall. "I'll meet you at home?" she asks, keeping step with him. "I wish we were in the same car. It's a nuisance, isn't it, always having to go separately?"

"Follow me," Bairstow says. "I want to show you something."

Miriam glances at him questioningly, but waits for him at the entrance of the parking lot. In a moment he pulls ahead, and with a wave, she follows. Bairstow turns away from their accustomed route home, to the park where June had led him, sliding into the same parking space he'd used so recently. This place is as lovely today as then, he thinks, with the shore stretching in a gentle curve away from them, and the waterfall opposite.

"It's...beautiful," exclaims Miriam, emerging from the car, looking out over the lake toward where the swans are grouped along the far shore. "How on earth did...?"

Bairstow comes to stand beside her. "For some reason, it isn't on the city map, Mimi, because I looked. Perhaps they haven't upgraded the maps since this was built. Or maybe the architect is trying to keep it for himself."

Miriam begins to walk toward the shore. "I wish I had some bread for the swans, Bairstow. Don't you? One day I'll bring some with me. The boys would love it...and Amanda, too, when she's better."

Miriam plans ahead for the family: Bairstow's always admired it in her. When she enjoys a thing, she wants it for others. But today the pond, at least for the moment, is theirs, as it was for Bairstow and June after they'd encountered Amanda in the restaurant. It's as if June had discovered a secret and has now passed it on to others who may be in need of a little beauty and peace.

"It's a place you want to stay forever," murmurs Miriam. "Shangri-La, almost in our own neighborhood. Was it June who showed it to you?"

Bairstow is taken by surprise; he feels the question as though it has a burning edge. "Yes. Does it make any difference?"

Miriam shakes her head, walking along slowly with her face toward the swans, away from him. "Of course not. I guess I'm just a little envious of anyone who could show you such a place. I wish she hadn't been the first with you here."

He smiles and takes her hand. "And now I've shown it to you, Miriam. It's a gift, isn't it? It's true, we'll pass it on to the rest of the family."

She stops still and looks at him. "Ben, I don't know if you realize that I love you. You remember when you asked me? I told you I did then, do you remember?"

Bairstow looks at Miriam, again surprised. "Of course, I know that. I never doubted it at all. Have you doubted me?" Somehow they seem naked, standing there, the two of them, watching the swans, talking about love.

She shakes her head. "I've been happy with you the twenty years we've been together, Ben. I mean, would you marry me again? Would you do it all over?"

He walks to her and touches a hand to her cheek. "I'd do it over in a minute, Mimi. I think we're part of the same soul...but we need separateness, too. Lately my life has been something I can't understand. I've been trying to evaluate it and I've come up short. I can't explain it. I've been in a funk, and I apologize. Sometimes I need air, like today. Amanda..."

"I know, Ben. I've made every effort to give you space." She walks a few steps, then turns back. "I couldn't live without you; I'm afraid that's the fact of it; I wouldn't know what to do if you weren't in my life. I guess that's the way it is, even if it sounds so...simple."

He catches her hand. "I feel the same, don't you know that?" He understands it, clearly and honestly, but perhaps he doesn't say so often enough, he doesn't take time to impress it on her. It's his failing, he doesn't do half the things he should anywhere near often enough. "Maybe I'd not survive without you, either, my dear. Why, Mimi," he says, "are you going to leave me for a younger man?"

The inconcongruity of it is so unbearable that Miriam's eyes fill with tears. "Oh, darling," she says, brushing them away. Then she laughs softly. "You are so...funny."

It's a help, Miriam's laughter, as if a dam has broken for both of them. When she stops, she grasps his arm again and they retrace their steps. "Ben, our lives are so...different. We are such different people that it's amazing how close we are in spite of it."

"Everyone is different," Bairstow answers. "But I'd say we're lots more similar than most." Then he stops suddenly, observing that three swans have gathered in their path. Bairstow steers Miriam clear, gently moving her to one side. "They're fierce birds," he says. "Do you remember when Tommy Craig's hand was broken by one on a trip to England when they got too close to a flock on the banks of the Thames?"

"I remember. "But we're clear of them. Still, they're magnificent creatures, aren't they?"

By the time they regain their cars, a few other people are arriving and ambling in the direction of the lake, some carrying bread for the swans. They wave as they pass each other along the path. Bairstow and Miriam are the only ones returning to the parking lot. "You're coming home now, Bairstow?" Miriam asks. "You don't have to return to the hospital?"

"I'll follow you," he answers. "I'll be right behind you."

She grasps his hand. "Thanks you for showing me this place. It's very special, isn't it?"

"Yes, it's special."

"Then I'll see you at home." She gives him a light kiss on the cheek, despite the fact that they will meet again in minutes. "To meeting at home," she says, raising her hand as if offering a mock toast.

Bairstow waits until Miriam has pulled forward in her car, then turns his to follow. She waves out the window and he waves back. .

At home the twins are playing softball in the backyard with some kids from the neighborhood. Bairstow remembers the kids vaguely. "Hey, Dad," Norman yells. "Play softball with us? We only got five. You c'n play outfield."

Bairstow turns: five faces are looking at him uncertainly, expectantly, hopeful that he'll round out their roster. What on earth makes them think I can play, much less want to play, softball? He certainly hasn't joined their game before. He starts to turn away, planning to yell back something like, "Sorry, kids, I'm on call," but on some impulse he stops still. How long has it been, he wonders idly, since I've played softball...or anything for that matter...with the kids? Why would they even think to ask me?

He turns slowly to Norman. "You got a mitt?" he asks to his own utter amazement. "And can you wait while I change my shoes?"

Both Norman and Pete are spurred to instant action.. "Great!" says Norman, "you mean it, Dad?" Pete without hesitation races into the garage for the mitt.

"What are you doing?" Miriam asks in surprise as her husband rushes through the kitchen, shedding his jacket on a chair as he goes.

"Playing ball, Mimi," he answers, barely turning his head. "They're letting me play outfield."

She hesitates, a cooking spoon suspended in her hand. "Letting you do *what*?"

"I can't stop to explain," he answers as he fetches his old shoes from the hall closet, then perches on the edge of a kitchen chair while he ties the laces. "My team desperately needs me on the diamond."

She stops, lacking an appropriate answer. "Ben," she says finally, "you're crazy, you know it?"

"Without a doubt, Mimi. Come and watch, I'm gonna need a cheering section." As he hurries out the kitchen door, he offers a brief salute to his astonished wife. Then he disappears.

It's a feeling he hasn't felt for a long while—this heady, headlong dash into competition, even if it's a mere backlot game with kids, two of them his own. He feels a little like a kid himself. Miriam actually comes out the back door to watch.

"You play out there," says one of the kids, not his own, pointing. "Out by the apple tree."

They think I don't know where the outfield is? he asks himself, mildly miffed. Why, I used to play on my college team, if they only knew, in the good old days shortly after the dinosaurs. He's on the team with Pete and a kid with carrot-top red hair. When a ball comes his way, he fumbles it.

"It's all right, Dad," says Pete kindly. "You'll get warmed up. Don't worry about it."

I'm *not* worried, Bairstow thinks, and when he comes up to bat, on the count of three balls and two strikes, on the brink of doom, he pastes the ball past the apple tree.

"You're a brick," yells the carrot-top kid. "Wow! Wow! Atta boy, Dr. Bairstow!"

"Super terrific, Dad, " yells Pete, jumping up and down. "Come on in! Come on in!" He's waving frantically.

He actually scores, leading Carrot-top to give him a high-five. Miriam has brought out a beach chair and is applauding. "I knew you could do it," she calls. "Yay, Ben. Yay, team!"

Bairstow feels amply vindicated. And he hasn't been called a boy in recent memory. "How'd you know my name?" he asks Carrot-top.

He points, "I live right over there. Pete's my friend."

"You're Herb Mathewson's boy?"

"Yep," he says. "Lionel."

Only Mathewson would name a kid Lionel, Bairstow reflects, but this is one nice kid.

An hour later, the game is ending and Miriam brings out brownies and passes them around. Mathewson, having heard the cheers from next door, has come over to watch. "Looks like you're having fun," Herb says, munching a brownie. "I didn't know you were such an athlete, Bairstow."

Bairstow laughs. "Maybe once," he says. "Now I spend too damn much time in the hospital. How are your flowers growing?"

"Good, since you told me how to make that mulch pile."

Miriam watches the two neighbors idly chatting and wonders what on earth has gotten into Ben? I haven't seen him have so much fun in years, she thinks. Why, he's positively turned into a..a…jock.

CHAPTER SIXTEEN

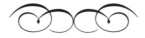

The next morning, before he can see Amanda, Bairstow receives the call for emergency surgery: another car accident. This time Potter is there to help, having finally returned from his weekend bicycle race in Connecticut. An older man has been injured and has gashes on his chest and neck where the windshield shattered and sliced his skin. His wife, thrown clear, is nevertheless undergoing surgery in another operating room of the hospital. The man has lost blood, but his repair is neither as extensive nor as grueling as that performed on Helen Proctor, Amanda, or presumably, Mario. This patient is merely anesthetized and requires stitching.

The rhythm of the operating room is once again established, and this time Potter is performing the surgery with Bairstow assisting. Potter appears subdued to Bairstow's eye, accustomed as he is to his assistant's moods. After a long interval when only the noises of the equipment sound throughout the room, Potter unexpectedly looks up from the knot he's tying. "June told me," he says.

"Told you?" Bairstow's eyebrows arch over his mask. "About what?"

"The growth. Maybe I should say malignancy in her lungs. It doesn't look good, does it?"

"You've seen the films?"

Potter nods. "This morning. I practically got Ebersole out of bed. In fact, I did. I couldn't believe it when June told me. Thanks, Bairstow."

"I didn't do anything, Potter. You'd have done the same for Miriam--if I were out of town."

Potter nods. "But you never go away, Bairstow. I do. All the time. It dawned on me. Maybe I'm away too damned much."

Bairstow bends again over his stitching. "Maybe that's the truth."

Potter stops moving the needle through the patient's torn flesh and looks archly back at Bairstow across the table. "What do you mean by that?"

Bairstow is trying to isolate a bleeder in the field before him, and for a moment can't answer. When he looks up, he finds Potter staring at him. "I didn't mean anything, Jeff. Let's talk it over when we're finished, all right?"

"No, Bairstow, I want to talk it over now."

Bairstow can see the anesthesiologist's head craning over the console: today; it's not Ferraro but his assistant, a man named Dever. The nurse stationed beside Potter glances apprehensively back and forth between the two men.

"There's nothing to talk about," says Bairstow. "Annie, will you please hold that retractor still."

The nurse rushes to comply, and Bairstow takes the needle holder from her.

"You're implying that I'm away too much," says Potter. "Is that it? At least that's what I interpret your silence to mean."

Bairstow takes a stitch. "Interpret it any way you wish, Potter. Let's talk later. Listen, we've got a job of work here..."

"Explain what you meant, Bairstow. Right now! I want to hear it."

Bairstow stands at full height now. "Get hold of yourself, Jeff. Are you all right? Listen, we can talk afterward, I already told you. Lord knows…"

"Well, you don't think I'm with June enough, that's it, isn't it? That's what it's all about. Why don't you just say so and get it over with?"

"Potter, stop it *now*. I don't know what your trouble is, but…"

"But what?"

Bairstow looks around. Dever is standing now, wary, worried. The nurse has been trying to retract the wound, but she hesitates, not knowing what will happen next. This, thinks Bairstow, is the last place in the world to be childish. "I'll ask you to leave surgery if you continue this way," Bairstow says. He knows that this is it, the end of their professional relationship if Potter doesn't get control of himself. He's never asked a man to leave the operating room before, and he's seen it happen only once, the time his colleague threw out an inebriated surgeon.

Potter drops the curved needle in its holder onto the floor and stalks from the room, flinging wide the heavy operating room door.

"Holy Jesus Christ, what was that about?" asks Dever. He leans over the console, looking stricken, his hand on top of his surgical cap as if to keep it from floating away.

"I'm not too sure myself," confesses Bairstow. "Let's finish this up so I can go talk to him."

"Well, I sure hope it doesn't happen again," says Dever. "You tell him for me I won't work with him if it does."

"It won't happen again," says Bairstow. "If it does, I won't work with him, either."

Bairstow has Potter paged as soon as he's through surgery, but the man doesn't answer. Yet Bairstow can see his car in the doctors' parking lot, so he must be around somewhere. Bairstow has a half-hour before his next case, so he sets out to find him. He's not in the doctors' office nor in the dressing rooms nor in the scrub area, either. His professional office is not in the hospital, as is Bairstow's, but three blocks away, and the chances are that if he'd gone to his office he'd have taken his car.

Bairstow finally locates him in the tiny cafeteria, having coffee by himself in a corner by the window. Bairstow helps himself to a cup, sets it on the tray with a glass of orange juice, and walks over to Potter's table. For a moment Potter glares at him as if he might hit him, or leave, or both. But he doesn't move, so Bairstow places his tray on Potter's table and pulls up a chair opposite.

"You aren't welcome," says Potter, looking away.

"I know that. But all the other tables are occupied."

Potter looks around: there isn't another person in the entire cafeteria.

Bairstow drinks his orange juice, then begins on his coffee. "Listen, Jeff, I wasn't criticizing the way you act with June," he says finally. "I don't even know how you act with June, and it's none of my business, anyway. But she's going through one terrible time. At least you know about that now. And when I think about it, I get pretty mad, too, because I feel you should have been here to help her out."

Potter glares at Bairstow again, setting his eyebrows into an angry, dark furl. "Well, old buddy, you *were* here, now weren't you? You seemed to fill in very nicely."

Bairstow places his fingertips together on the table before him. "I don't know what the trouble is, Jeff. For *your* information, my daughter's been in an automobile accident. Two died and the other's probably not going to make it. Amanda's in traction. In the meantime, June needed help. She needed support, and she's my patient. You weren't here and you should have been."

For the first time, Potter glances over at Bairstow. He shakes his head slowly and his anger seems to dissipate. His jaw drops. "Amanda? You mean it?"

Bairstow looks at the younger man. "You think I'm joking?"

"I...didn't know, Bairstow. Jesus! I spoke with June about twenty minutes this morning—then I beat it over to find Ebersole. I didn't hear about Amanda. How is she?"

Bairstow stirs his coffee. "Amanda's coming along. Miriam's with her now."

Potter readjusts himself, extending his elbows onto the table. "So I guess...you're still telling me that I'm not taking care of June properly?" His jaw sets once again into a tight line.

"Of course I'm not saying any such thing. But she needs you, Potter. That's the truth. I don't know what's going on with her health, but it frankly doesn't look good. It could be lots of things. You know she's coming in for another scan today?"

He nods. "Ten o'clock. I've canceled out everything else on my calendar. Kulick's going to take my case--he'll be assisting you."

Bairstow smiles. "I'm glad you warned me."

Potter looks more intently at Bairstow, and this time his eyes are almost pleading. "What do you think, Ben...about June, I mean? You're her docter. Tell me..."

Bairstow hardly thinks about it, that in private comversations such as this, the men call each other by their first names, but during working hours they each refer to the other by last names. This is first-name time.

Bairstow shoves his coffee away. "I don't know, honestly, Jeff. Tumor, yes. Malignant? I don't know. We'll know a lot more after the scan and the biopsy. Operable? Who knows--we'll have to see where it lies. We'll have to go step by step."

Their relationship has suddenly shifted, Bairstow can feel it. In his own need, Potter has turned into a supplicant, as Amanda has done in her crisis. His outburst in the operating room has a great deal to do with June, but much to do with Potter himself, who's having trouble coping with his own feelings. Bairstow can remember his own immaturities in the past, and understands very well that a skilled surgeon often isn't gifted in human relationships: June has taught him a little and Miriam a great deal in this department. He's older than Potter and the younger man has turned to him.

"You'll meet with me later?" Potter asks. "After June's gone through the scan?"

"If you want me to. I'll check in after my surgery."

Potter moves his hand across his forehead. "I'm damned sorry, Bairstow. I don't know what the hell is wrong with me lately."

Bairstow stands up to leave, placing his hand on Potter's shoulder. "Forget it, Jeff. We all have bad days." Yet for some reason Bairstow feels a resurgence of energy despite the sleepless night, despite Amanda's accident and Jeff's blowup. Maybe it's because Amanda's alive, or perhaps it's because Miriam loves him. It may be because of June: her composure and quiet strength refresh him. He hurries up the stairs, ignoring the elevator. When he enters Amanda's room, she's awake, seeming relaxed against the pillows, yet overshadowed by the structure of her leg pulley. "Hi," she says. "It's funny, but I knew you'd come. In fact, I knew you'd come now. It's almost as if I willed it."

June had said the same thing when he arrived unexpectedly at her house, an odd coincidence. Bairstow chuckles. "Maybe you've become psychic after your accident, Amanda. Strange things happen with trauma."

"I doubt it, but anyway I'm glad you came. By the way, who *was* that woman I saw you with at lunch that day? She was very attractive."

He can refuse to tell her—it's really none of her business--but he has no reason to keep it a secret from her. "Jeff Potter's wife. She may have a very serious illness. We'd just come from the hospital."

"But she looked all right to me."

Bairstow notices that since he's last seen his daughter, her cast has been thoroughly autographed with pictures, verse and exclamation points in a multitude of colors. "I hope she's all right, Amanda. She's having more tests today."

Amanda studies her father's face for a moment. "I guess I was pretty...rude that day. Sorry. If I was rude, I mean."

"That's not what June said. She thought I was rude. I'm afraid she thinks I'm unfeeling sometimes. I've been trying to change my habits."

It takes a moment for Bairstow's words to settle on his daughter. Her face shifts through the varying emotions of the process: disbelief to thoughtfulness, to rapt attention. "She must be pretty interesting," Amanda ventures.

"She is."

"Does mother know about her?"

Bairstow looks full at her face. "What's there to know? Don't you think you're being a little silly?"

Amanda shifts in the bed. "I won't tell. Did you know that Mario is only a casual friend? Well, actually he started as a friend of a friend. He loaned my friend money."

Bairstow is afraid he can see the outlines of the situation. "For drugs? Is that what the money was for?"

Amanda moves her finger along the edge of the mattress. "Yes, but my friend was in debt. She passed a check which bounced, but it really wasn't her fault because her parents were supposed to have deposited the tuition money into that account. They didn't, and when she got uppity, they said they wouldn't give her a cent. So she turned to Mario--and he said he'd get it for her."

"For a price, I bet."

"For sure. I know, it was a bad scene. You won't believe it, but I was going to tell them I didn't want anything to do with them even if the woman was a friend. Except they'd invited me to lunch to talk about it, and I accepted. My friend was going home--and Mario was heading back to his place."

Bairstow can feel the dislike of the scene Mario represents, but he doesn't want to get into an argument with Amanda, nor tell her how absurd he thinks she is to be dealing with those people. Besides, she seems to already know it. And she almost got killed. "And then later you had the accident."

"Yes. We were all going...to see someone else."

A sudden thought occurs to Bairstow. "Amanda, was Mario involved in any way in your shoplifting?"

She nods slowly. "We gave what we stole to Mario to help pay for the loan. He disposed of it. Pretty silly because that was the first and last time I stole. I got caught because I was so bad at it, and I made twelve dollars total. Eileen made forty, and she didn't get caught."

The story makes Bairstow feel depressed. He can't imagine what Miriam will say when she hears it, but he suspects that she'll cry. At least Amanda has been honest with him. Maybe it would have made a difference with the judge, that she had not committed grand theft, although stealing is stealing no matter what the amount. At least, please good God, maybe she won't do it again.

"I have another case coming right up," Bairstow says. "I'll be back, Amanda. Are you feeling all right?"

"Stiff," she says. "I feel like an idiot with my leg this way. It aches like crazy."

"Do you want something for it?"

She shakes her head. "I don't want anything. I'll be all right."

"We'll bring you a pizza tonight if you want one. The boys can get it for you." He smiles archly. "Or do you prefer hospital food?"

She makes a face. "You've got to be joking!"

Bairstow returns to his office, to reread the last notes he's placed on the chart before surgery on his patient now in the hospital. She has a lump in her breast, suspected to be cancerous by mammogram and biopsy. Bairstow will assist the plastic surgeon for the breast reconstruction. To Bairstow, such planning makes sense--if he were a woman he'd do the same thing. Strange, he thinks, that in the old days of his training, entire breasts and their underlying muscles were excised at the least hint of cancer; but of course they had no radiation therapy then.

As he enters his office, even before switching on his light, he can see a form, then realizes that it's a large rectangular box. Without even having to wonder, he knows instantly what it is: June's picture, wrapped in sheets of cardboard amd covered with a heavy cloth. Good God, he thinks, she's giving it to me; she really meant it. What did I do to warrant this enormous gift? I don't really deserve it. He feels thunderstruck as he very carefully unwraps the large frame, discards the coverings, props it against his desk, then stands back to look at it.

Even in the semi-dark it's an astonishingly beautiful painting. June paints in curves separating the vivid colors into zones which enhance each other and coalesce in the observer's eye. Onto that background she paints simply, vividly, with skill and control. This picture she has given him is his favorite, the bentwood chairs before an ocean of deep, luminous blue and a stylized background of vivid flowers balancing the chairs and presided over by a distant nude figure reclining on a chaise. Bairstow can almost see, hear and touch June in the canvas, so much of her is in it. Yet he doubts that anyone else can see it, perhaps even Potter. Here is her warmth and vividness and verve. He would never confuse her style with that of another painter, because hers has its own distinction. It's a gift of herself, that's what it is--and she always gives of herself. When he places this picture on his wall, he will always see June in it.

He covers it again and reties the wraps firmly--he'd rather not see it again until he places it on the wall of his living room. But then, he doesn't know how Miriam will accept it but thinks she will take it with astonishment and awe in the same spirit of friendship with which it was given.

He arrives at surgery only to find that the Goldman case is holding up the queue of patients on today's operating schedule. Goldman has arranged a facelift for one of his female patients, and the woman seems to be bleeding abnormally for some reason which didn't come to light in pre-operative testing, so Goldman's taking unusual pains, which translate into time. At least that's what Kulick reports. Kulick is barely five-and-a-half feet tall, a sawed-off, belligerent kind of man whom

Potter describes as having a "little man complex." When Bairstow heard the term before, he discounted it as pseudo-psychiatric jargon, but if there really is such a thing, he supposes Kulick has it. Kulick's a good surgeon, at least. Patients don't like him very well, so he assists other men frequently, as he is with Bairstow today, and covers their practices when they're away. Kulick is pacing the floor, peering from time to time through the window into the operating room to see what progress Goldman is making.

"Do you think that guy will *ever* finish?" he fumes. "Can you imagine the agony of it? I mean, his damned little stitches take hours, along with all his fussing around, hemming and hawing." Kulick is running his hands through his stubby straight hair, waiting to tie on his surgical cap.

"Try brain surgery," says Bairstow, thinking of Mario and the delicate maneuvering Plotkin performed on him over at the Center, all those hours while they picked bone fragments from his brain.

"*You* think of brain surgery," says Kulick with a snort. "I'd rather not. All that finicky stuff would drive me nuts."

Bairstow reflects that on a regular basis, it *would* drive Kulick nuts--but he's also seen the man spend inhuman and agonizing periods of time digging around human insides to find leaks in ventral valves and in veins where stitches have mysteriously blown. Despite his blather, Kulick is one of the most finicky men Bairstow knows in the surgical arena. They stand around waiting it out until Goldman, sweating with the effort and the confining layers of the operating gown, joins them; the patient has already disappeared into the adjacent recovery area.

"Sorry," Goldman says, mopping his face, "I didn't know she was a bleeder. Someone's gonna have his ass kicked when I get through with him. Where in God's name do you suppose they got the blood coagulation test that I read?"

It's an old story to Bairstow that tests in hospitals get mixed up, that sometimes they aren't performed correctly, and sometimes they aren't performed at all. He himself has railed at laboratory chiefs and technicians alike, and even managed to get a few fired. For some ungodly reason, in his opinion, hospital administrators, who continually draw the ire of physicians for their narrow-minded, money-conscious mishandling of hospitals affairs, tend nevertheless to protect careless people unconscionably because usually they're hired by the hospital administration itself. He has a basic distrust of hospital directors because in his opinion they could care less about the innocent victims of their penny-pinching: patients. But now his patient is being moved in, so Kulick and Bairstow hurriedly complete the scrubbing and gowning, and walk together into the operating room.

A half-hour later, the surgery is over just as Bairstow had anticipated, with no need for Goldman's expertise: the tumor is benign and requires merely simple removal. As he closes the woman's breast, he is thinking of June, knowing that she must be undergoing the CT scan about this time. He feels anxious and unsettled about it--but at least this time Potter is with her. He even feels apprehensive about Potter, not knowing if the man can cope: he's seen the man come apart today. But he's *got* to cope, he *must* give comfort to his wife, there's no other way. Perhaps for the first time in his life Potter must really extend himself to those who need him. Bairstow hopes for the best; he himself will be there if he's needed, but just maybe Potter will hold up this time. There's always hope.

CHAPTER SEVENTEEN

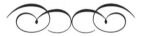

The CT scan is still in progress when Bairstow threads his way through the subterranean hospital corridors and ends up in radiology. A receptionist tells him that June is still in the long, cylindrical donut in the next wing. The machine is gobbling her up inch by inch and transposing her into core shavings, like the cross section of a tree. The mass in her chest is being pictured as a series of slices, which Ebersole reads precisely and will present as findings to Bairstow when the diagnostic work is done, when the machine has had its fill and expelled its patient like Jonah from the whale. Bairstow has never bothered to decipher the peculiar tracings of the complicated machine: they are the expertise of others, and he has his own domain in which he must remain proficient. There is already too much diversity in medicine these days, he thinks, to go dabbling very far afield.

Potter is perched on one of the unconscionably uncomfortable chairs in Ebersole's front parlor, nervous as a twit.

"How long has it been going on?" asks Bairstow. "Can I get you a cup of coffee, Jeff?"

Potter shakes his head. "I'd get sick," he says. "I threw my cookies a half-hour ago."

Bairstow knows how the man feels: he still can't cloak himself in a feeling of neutrality about this case, either, as he usually can in touchy, unclear situations. He has a sense of foreboding, of unease. Damn, he thinks once again, why doesn't Ebersole fix up this place so that at least you have light to read by? Why must slats from the chair seat stick you in the rear end when you're dealing with the trauma of someone you care about undergoing tests which determine life or death? Why doesn't Ebersole sink some of his hospital-donated money into the care and nurturing of patients' families as well as monster machines?

Bairstow tries to engage Potter in conversation, asking him once again about his bicycle trip, not that Bairstow is particularly interested, but hoping it will distract Jeff from his funk. "I can't talk about it," says Potter, looking embarrassed. "I can't even remember it."

So there's nothing to do but agonize. Bairstow tries to read a three-month-old magazine detailing the life of one of the latest emerging nubile starlets who apparently fought for the privilege of bedding down with a noted producer as the best route to further her career. He throws that one down and picks up another, an article about the ravaged and disappearing genus of American elk. Then he puts that one aside, too. He's as bad as Potter, he can't remember what he's reading, even though he'd like to know about the elk. But neither of them has long to wait because within five minute Ebersole appears through the closed door from the direction of his CT room. Ebersole looks around: it's a delicate moment, because Bairstow is the referring physician but Potter's the husband. Bairstow immediately defers to Potter as he knows Potter would to him should the patient in the next room have been Miriam.

Ebersole's the only one in the room not depressed: he's even buoyant as always, but then he's trained to present his findings to other doctors, not to worried patients. Which is lucky, Bairstow's always thought, because the man has a terrible bedside manner; in fact, he has none at all; he's as cold as last winter's squash.

"Well, there's a mass, all right," says Ebersole. "Right anterior lobe. I'll show you when the tracings are ready."

"How big?" asks Potter.

"Can't tell you this moment for sure, but it's wedged in between the sternum and the third and fourth ribs. About ten centimeters, I'd estimate, but I'll know for sure..."

It sounds like a grim sentence to Bairstow. He attempts to speak in Ebersole's matter-of-fact tone, but can't make it, even for Potter's sake. "Is it operable?" he manages to ask Ebersole.

Ebersole shrugs. "Don't see why not. Better get in there pretty fast, though, before it gets any larger. Are you contemplating radiation and chemotherapy?" The question is directed toward Potter.

"I don't know," Potter says. He's coming apart again; Bairstow can see the symptoms: his hands are trembling slightly and his face, previously flushed, is turning pale, as if he might faint. "We'll talk to the oncologists," says Bairstow. "I'll handle it, Ebersole."

Ebersole nods: Potter's distress is obvious. "All right. Let me know how you decide to handle the radiation, I'll sick Mendino onto it." Mendino is a partner of Ebersole's who does therapeutic radiation under the direction of the oncologists, whose expertise in cancer treatment is required in cases like this.

"Jesus," says Potter, holding his head. "Holy Mother of God."

The door to the next room opens again, and a nurse enters. She approaches Potter with a smile. "Mrs. Potter will be right out, Dr. Potter. She says to wait, please."

Bairstow feels almost as limp as Potter. But by the time he manages to control his tumbling emotions, June is coming through the door, looking cool and smiling and elegant. She doesn't know, Bairstow is thinking, they haven't told her yet.

"Hi," she says. "I'm sorry if I kept you waiting."

Potter looks at her as if he's watching a mirage. "H...how are you?" he asks her. "Are you all right?"

"Of course. They put you in this big machine which looks like something right out of a science fiction movie. I never saw anything like it before." She smiles, embarrassed. "But I don't know why I'm describing it to you, when you already know." She turns to Ebersole. "Can I leave now? I mean, is there anything else I must do?"

Ebersole shakes his head. "Not now, but..." He glances at Bairstow.

"No, nothing else," says Bairstow, trying to squelch any comments Ebersole might make about further treatment before June fully understands her own condition. "I'll see you later, Max."

Ebersole nods at Potter. "You're heading home?"

"Yes." Potter stares at Bairstow. "Have we more cases? I don't seem to remember..."

Bairstow shakes his head. "Don't worry about it, Jeff. If anything turns up, I'll get someone else."

"No." Potter is very firm. "I have office hours later. I'll be here. Tell Martha I'll be here, will you?" Martha is Potter's office nurse.

"Sure," Bairstow answers. "Don't worry about it."

They're dressed in their jackets now. June turns back toward Bairstow and places her hand in his. "Thanks," she says. Her eye meets his and she smiles. "Thanks so much, Ben. For everything." Then she's gone, through the winding corridors trailed by Potter. For a moment Bairstow looks after her, wishing he could follow, to say words of comfort or consolation even if she doesn't yet know why. At least Potter is here, it's now his responsibility. He hasn't thanked her for the painting, but this is definitely not the time

Bairstow turns back to Ebersole. "I'll check the operating schedule and let you know, Max. About the surgery, I mean." They both understand that it is June's surgery under discussion. Radioactive procedures and scans will fall into Ebersole's domain and he must be informed as well. "First," Bairstow goes on, "Potter will have to tell his wife, and, for him, that will be the hard part."

Ebersole shrugs and picks up June's chart. "But she already knows."

"She *knows*? Who told her?"

"I did. She wanted to know. In fact, she insisted."

"But...how did she take it?"

"Without batting an eye. I told her she should have immediate surgery, that you'd undoubtedly say the same thing because it was her best chance."

He should have anticipated Ebersole's error: it was for Bairstow to drop the bombshell to June because he was her attending physician, or for Potter, but certainly not the chief of radiology. But the fact that Ebersole had blundered where he had no business angered but didn't surprise Bairstow, who knew him to be obtuse and downright insensitive on occasion. He'd remind Ebersole vigorously of this point of protocol at the next opportunity so the radiologist wouldn't waylay any more of his patients with unexpected diagnostic shocks.

June's courage also doesn't surprise him; of course that's the way she would act. If Potter were more of a man and could hold himself together, he would go to her now and comfort her, to help her through the difficulties ahead. Potter must rise to the occasion, and, who knows, Bairstow has reminded himself again, just maybe he will.

He calls Vicki Lane, the nurse in charge of operating room scheduling. "What have you got this week?" he asks. "Mrs. Potter will need an operating room as soon as possible."

She consults a long list. "Dr. Bairstow, you must live right or something because until ten minutes ago there wasn't a thing. We just had a concellation because Dr. Abernathy sent his hysterectomy home when she caught the flu." Once Bairstow had objected to the fact that hospital patients are, more often than not, designated by their diseases rather than their names, but at least he's learned to live with it.

"You're the admitting physician?" she asks.

"Yes, but someone else will do the surgery."

"Who's going to do it?"

Bairstow feels the air charged with her question. "Not Potter, for obvious reasons."

"For sure, boss. He's the husband, natch."

He's used to her flip remarks on occasion but likes Vicki and doesn't object. "But I'll be damned if I know who I'll get, Vicki. I'll call Kulick...and Snyder and McIntyre. We'll find someone."

"Well, Dr. Kulick's going to Bermuda, and Dr. McIntyre's at a medical meeting. I don't know about Dr. Snyder. You aren't doing it, Dr. Bairstow?"

"I'm too involved with the case, and I may be busy. I'll try Snyder and get back to you."

Bairstow ignores Vicki's pause--she can think what she wants about his involvement. But he's forgotten about Kulick's trip, the man told him weeks ago. Snyder is good, but he's new to the hospital, an unknown quantity. Bairstow walks back to his office, then calls Potter at home because it won't wait: if he's going to get the case onto the schedule, he's got to act right away. For a moment he hopes that June will answer, but Potter's voice is on the line. "Potter," he says, "you already know that June's growth must be removed as soon as possible. Ebersole doesn't like the look of it. It needs to come out."

His voice sounds despondent. "I know. June already told me."

"All right." Bairstow tries to keep his voice level. "How do you feel about Snyder as surgeon-in-chief?"

"Snyder?" Potter's voice cracks with impatience. "Are you kidding? Why won't you do it?"

"Because I'm your partner. I honestly don't think it's right...I'm close to both of you.."

"So what does being my partner have to do with it? I wouldn't *take* anyone else. June wouldn't, either. She already told me that."

"She...told you? She said that?"

"I wouldn't tell you if she hadn't."

"Where is she, Potter? Is she all right?"

"Sure. She's out for a spin. She said she'd be back in a while."

⸜⸝

Bairstow knows exactly where she's gone. He hurries into his car and drives as fast as he dares to the park. He can see her car there already, but he'd known all along, as if he had a mental photograph, where he'd find it. Nevertheless, it takes him ten minutes to spot her. She's sitting on a bench near a turn in the river; she's brought along bread to feed the swans.

"I knew you'd come," she says, not looking up. "I knew it, Ben. I swear we're telepathic." She looks up at him. "Thanks for coming, my dear."

"June, I have to talk to you. Doctors don't operate on their own families or those too close. I honestly don't know what to do. If there were anyone else available on short notice with surgical privileges at this hospital, I'd bring him in. Perhaps someone from Center would come over."

She looks up into his face. "I won't take anyone but you, Ben. I couldn't stand it. I'd prefer to die untreated if you won't help me."

Her response is an unexpected shock. She reaches forward and grasps his wrist. Farther down the path a couple is strolling; the woman looks back, hearing June's insistent words. But June is oblivious. "Say you will, Ben. You said you'll be there for me."

"And Potter?"

"He absolutely agrees. Dr. Ebersole, too. He called to give Jeff a walking tour of my body now that the CT scan is finished, and I told him I absolutely wanted you for my surgeon. See, I have you boxed in."

He looks at her searchingly, at the determined tilt of her chin. "All right, June. How can I refuse? But I'm not comfortable with it."

June turns limp and falls against him. "Thank you, Ben. Thank you so much. If anyone can cure me, you can. I feel that strongly."

They walk slowly around the side of the lake. He takes her hand. "Thanks for the picture. I forget to tell you. It's magnificent."

"It's to remember me by, no matter what happens. It's part of me, Ben--of our time together. You can consider it that way."

"I already do."

Bairstow's heart feels leaden: he must treat June as any other patient, as if she were someone he barely knew except in a medical capacity. That's what he's been dreading all along, the pain of it. Except that Potter is essential to this process, too, to explain to June the procedures, the preparations, what they are trying to accomplish, to ease along the recovery. Bairstow would do that, but now Potter must. He calls Potter's office during the afternoon and tells Martha that the case is scheduled for 9:00 a.m. on Thursday. "All right," says Martha, "I'll pass it on to him, but he's having a tough time."

"He isn't the only one."

In midafternoon, Bairstow cancels his appointments, telling Jan Valenti that he's going home, that she can take the rest of the afternoon off.

"Tough about Mrs. Potter," says Jan. "I found out about it through the grapevine. I hope you don't mind that I know."

"I rather think Mrs. Potter would be pleased."

"That's good, Dr. Bairstow. I hear she's a nice woman. I don't know how one faces that kind of thing."

"I don't either, Jan. I hope neither of us has to find out."

He stops to see Amanda, but she's asleep. Miriam has been there, the nurses tell Bairstow, that they played rummy together for an hour. "They used the cast to hold the cards," one nurse reports.

Bairstow laughs and turns away: Amanda is making progress, and for that he's thankful.

He returns to the office, removes his white coat, and sits before June's canvass for a while. It imparts her strength to him, he can't say how or why, but it does. He drives home more slowly than he can remember, causing a couple of drivers to honk at him; surprising, because he's usually the one who honks. He barely feels like moving, as if he's mired in quicksand. At home he removes the canvass from the car and carries it into the house. No one is there: the twins are in school, and Mirium is out somewhere, perhaps shopping or tending to her own affairs.

Bairstow finds a hammer in his toolbox in the garage, then carries the canvass along with the hammer into the living room. There, he sinks butterfly hooks into the frame to hold the mounting wire, then attaches the carved, gilt frame to the wall over the fireplace. Afterward, he stands back to better observe June's gift.

Color, he thinks, seems to radiate from the canvas, causing the dark room to pulse with life. Hues of green, maroon and gold blazing from the painting virtually set the living room to vibrating, as he knew they would. Until this moment, he had not fully realized what a truly beautiful room his architect had fashioned in this old house. We must entertain here, he thinks, this place has been empty too long. The twins will have to find some other place to roughhouse.

He has finished and stands in a trance admiring the canvas when he hears Miriam's step at the door and her footsteps as she enters the kitchen. In a minute he can hear her looking for him. "In here," he calls. She enters the room, then comes to him and circles his waist with her arm, gazing up at the painting.

"Oh, Ben," she says after a moment, "it's perfectly lovely. Why, this room is made for it. It makes all the difference..."

Bairstow nods and slips his arm about her.

"I assume it's June's. I saw her painting over the mantel at her house. I think I'd know her style anywhere, it's so sunny and vibrant."

"She wanted us to have it, Mimi."

"She wanted *you* to have it, Ben."

"You approve...?"

"Of course I approve. She's not only a nice person...but a talented painter besides." A thought occurs to her. "Then the tests..."

"Positive. We have to remove the tumor."

"Are *you* going to do it?"

"I don't want to but there's no one else. And I'm her doctor."

"But that's such a heavy responsibility."

"Yes."

"I'll pray for the best, Ben. I hope I'm not too rusty for prayer."

Bairstow kisses Miriam's hair at the top of her head, where there's a little cowlick. "I'm sure you're not, Mimi. I think if anyone's got influence, you do."

CHAPTER EIGHTEEN

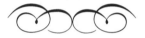

On Thursday, the rain comes down in torrential downpours, and Bairstow has to skirt puddles to reach the hospital on the main road by 6:30 a.m. Residents of Tennafield have been warned by the morning news to stay home until the cloudburts have ceased, that there might be danger of tornadoes before noon. Bairstow ignores all warnings because he must--and because he's a fatalist at heart, anyway. He feels that if he's killed he'll be dead and beyond worry; if he isn't, it's business as usual, and that involves surgery beginning this morning at 7:00 a.m . June's case is scheduled at 9:00. Today he's earlier than usual because he wants to read June's test reports again. Of course he's already double and triple checked them, but he can't afford to miss anything. He wants a picture in his mind of what he's going to encounter during surgery to minimize surprises. Surprises can be lifethreatening at worst and unsettling at best--and with June, particularly with June, he wants none of either.

When he enters June's room, she is sitting in bed looking scared. Her hair is tied in a ribbon, and she appears no older than Amanda.

She grasps his hand when he sits down beside her, and he feels no qualm that Potter will see them this way if he should enter now. This is a solemn moment for both, and Bairstow has sat this way with many patients before June, trying to impart strength and courage for what may lie ahead.

"I want you to know, Ben," she says, "that if anything should go wrong, I won't hold it against you. Even if I were to ultimately die from this cancer. You don't need to tell me how tricky some surgery can be..."

Bairstow takes her hand reassuringly between his. "I can almost guarantee that nothing will go wrong with the surgery, June. We have the best of facilities here, and you're healthy. The tumor on the second series of tests didn't look as formidable as on the first. It will just take a little time to recover..and patience." In his own ears he can hear the speech he gives to most patients, and he wishes he didn't have such damnable self-knowledge because he wants it fresh for her ears alone. Yet he is speaking medical truths and good sense.

She looks back at him, her blue eyes wide and fixed on his face. "I don't mean that you aren't a wonderful surgeon, either, Ben. Jeff says you're the best there is, and I already know that's true."

"June..." he begins, but she interrupts again.

"And," she says, a little breathlessly, "I don't want you to think that...because of the other day in my studio, I mean...I have any hold over you or anything. You understand that, don't you?"

Bairstow, touched, leans forward and can clearly see that her eyes are becoming slowly dilated from the pre-surgery drugs, designed to alleviate her anxiety. She leans back against the pillow. "I never thought you intended any hold over me, June. It was a gesture of...tenderness, a special time. Now allow yourself to fall asleep. The nurses will be with you in a minute."

"I *do* sound a little off the track, don't I? What's in those pills they gave me? I want to tell you about Jeff before I fall asleep, Ben--he's doing so much better. What did you say to him--he's..."

As he holds her hand, her eyes flutter and close as he's watching. It was not going to be an easy morning for either of them.

"Damn bloody, going into chests," says Snyder to no one in particular. Snyder is assisting Bairstow, having been called into action for this surgery before departing for a week's vacation. "You've got all that vascularized tissue." June is lying on her side, anesthetized, with a table of instruments swung out over her head. Just now, no one is aware of her as a breathing, functioning human with a personality except Bairstow, who's fighting it to attain detached judgment. A section of rib cage shows through the draping, slathered with Betadine orange to ward off infection. Bairstow has already begun below June's breast, cutting not with an ordinary knife but with an electric scalpel along the contour of a rib, ending halfway down the left side of her back. "This should sear through the small blood vessels," Bairstow says in response to Snyder's remark about the blood. "There'll be less blood this way." He's not used to operating with Snyder, and his tensions are already high, but he wants to accommodate the man within reason. And talking aloud as he goes helps him focus. "There," he points out, "is the latissimus dorsi, you can make it out." Bairstow must speak more loudly than usual so his voice will carry over the sparking of the electric scalpel, which emits an annoying buzz like an errant bee, but at least it does its job.

"Yes...I see it," says Snyder. "Here, hand me that retractor." He turns to the young nurse beside him, an assistant he's brought along to this surgery: Snyder has explained that she's taking six months of operative nursing at the completion of her training and this case will complete the course.

Bairstow puts two rubber-clad fingers beneath the wide muscles of June's back, easing, as gently as he can, the muscles away from the underlying tissue. As the blood oozes, Snyder stitches the tear. Thank God, he's good, Bairstow thinks as he watches the man lay down stitches with precision; this surgery won't take so long with competent assistance and June won't be under anesthetic for so long. He'd originally allowed four hours on the schedule, but can now hope for not much more than three if all goes well.

"This is the rhomboid muscle, attached to the scapula," Bairstow explains to the young nurse. The second nurse is again Charlotte Kirkham. Bairstow moves to the other end of the incision. "And that's the serratur muscle." Bairstow is moving the muscle to one side. He's busy, moving quickly but surely now, in familiar territory, at ease. He knows where he's going, and that settles him.

"They can really *cure* this kind of tumor?" the young nurse asks, her voice betraying her doubt.

"Certainly," Bairstow reassures her. "More often than not."

Snyder agrees, the words muffled by his mask. "Lots of people walking around town cured of cancer, young lady."

"I know but..." The young nurse doesn't finish her sentence but glances over at Bairstow and points to the instrument Charlotte has just handed him. "What are you going to do with *that*, Dr. Bairstow?"

Snyder glances at Bairstow to see if he's objecting to this sort of questioning, but Bairstow shakes his head with a barely imperceptible movement. "We must remove a rib, this time the fifth rib." He eases the chisel through the cartilage and severs the rib as Charlotte holds back the surrounding tissue.

"See," says Snyder with a laugh, "a spare rib. Don't you like spare ribs and sauerkraut?"

It's another one of the senseless, tasteless operating room jokes, and today it makes Bairstow angry. Yet he keeps his eyes focused on the field, ignoring the comment. But the young nurse giggles and Charlotte Kirkham laughs aloud.

Now Bairstow can see the lung, a purple, shiny mass. So far, so good, Bairstow thinks, reaching his hand, knuckles up, through the slot in June's chest. He slides his fingers far up along the inside of the chest wall toward whatever it is that made the shadow on the scan. He feels it. "God," he exclaims, almost unaware that he's said it. "This tumor has gone up into the chest wall."

Snyder nods grimly, and neither of the nurses says anything. Bairstow is relieved that at least June can't hear his words because they sound not only forbidding but also like a verdict. Yet there's hope still; he'll fight for every glimmer. "The rib spreader," says Bairstow, holding out his hand, still examining the dark space inside June's body where the tumor has lodged itself.

He positions the machine between the fourth and sixth ribs and cranks: slowly more space becomes available, and he can extend his hand farther into the lung area. "It's operable," he says almost triumphantly, still feeling the slippery mass of the lung with the tumor encroached on it. "But it's in a bad position, right over the aorta." He turns to the anesthesiologist, a part-time staff man named Christiansen, who hasn't said a word, but sits with his eyes fastened on the console readings. "Have you got enough blood, Dave?"

"Luckily," the man answers. "I'm ready for anything, Ben. Want me to start the first unit?"

Bairstow nods, and when he sees that blood is dripping steadily into June's veins, he cuts again, this time deeply into the tumor area. It's up to him now: whatever happens to June is in his hands. The powers that be may control the growth of the tumor, but at this moment he controls its removal. He focuses on the area, drawing Snyder and the nurses into the assault. "I need to go in here distally," he explains. "Hand me the clip to remove the growth, Charlotte. She'll get radiation so we've got to excise every bit of malignant tissue." He examines the area. "See that patch here...and there, Snyder. Let's go for it."

"I see it, Bairstow. I'm with you."

Bairstow is so intense he feels almost feverish. "The artery's in good shape. Thank God for small favors."

"You'll remove the lobe?" Snyder asks, not looking up.

Bairstow nods. "Without it she'll stand X-ray therapy better."

Later, in a moment of reflection, Snyder stands back from the table. "Hell of a lot of tumor," he says. "What do you think, Bairstow?"

Bairstow hasn't shifted position in the last half-hour. Nothing, not the sound of pessimism in Snyder's voice or his own self-doubt will deter him from this struggle. "We'll remove it," he says. "How's she doing?" he asks the anesthesiologist.

"Okay, Bairstow. Normal beat. All signs normal." They can hear the rhythm of June's heart throughout the room: ta-dah. ta-dah. ta-dah." It reassures Bairstow. "Have you any 3-0?" The young nurse hands him the suture material deftly, and he begins to stitch. The minutes and hours are passing on the wall clock, shooting Bairstow's time estimate to oblivion. Finally Bairstow turns to the anesthesiologist. "Hyperventilate the patient, please." He spills a jug of saline solution about the interior of the body cavity, watching for bubbles of air which might indicate a leakage. Then he drains the chest and closes.

The young nurse, no matter how many cases she's seen, is shocked. "But isn't she going to feel a terrible lot of pain, Dr. Bairstow? I mean, how long will it take her to recover?"

"She'll stay in the hospital for a while," Bairstow answers. "The pain is variable, person-to-person. This woman has remarkable courage, so I think she'll handle it well. She'll recover quickly."

The young nurse is overcome with curiosity. "Just what do you call this operation," she persists across the table despite Charlotte's pointed glances. "Does it have a name?"

"Of course," Snyder answers, coming to Bairstow's rescue. "It's called a right upper lobectomy. Don't ask so many questions, please, when the surgery is still going on."

"I'm sorry," the nurse answers, but Bairstow smiles at her. "That's how you learn. Please hand me another suture."

They help to undrape June and transfer her from the table to the gurney. She's so very beautiful, Bairstow thinks as he looks at her: her head is back with her small chin thrust upward. Her soft hair is spread about her face like a halo. Her surgery is over and he has done his level best; now he must explain to Potter what he's found.

Potter is outside the door, pacing like a caged animal. Bairstow removes his operating cap and leads him to a chair in a quiet corner. "Jesus, it took a while," he says. "My God, Bairstow, what happened in there?"

"Sit down, Jeff, June's all right. We removed a lobe, pretty extensive, more than we bargained for..."

Potter grasps his arm. "But will she recover? Tell me! What do you think?"

Baistow looks reassuringly at him. "Get yourself together, man. She'll do all right, I think. With your support and good judgment..."

Potter nods and rubs his head apologetically. "Sorry. I'm making a damned ass of myself."

"You're naturally worried..."

"I'm a pain in the butt, Bairstow. Don't give up on me, all right?"

Bairstow claps his hand on Potter's shoulder. "I'm a lousy stoic myself, Jeff. And no one's giving up on you"

"I just don't want her hurt. I don't want her to die. Please God..."

"She's not going to die, Jeff. With radiation, I think she'll do fine. You've got to think positively and forget your negative thoughts."

"Sorry. Of course I'll try." He takes a breath. "Did I tell you that June and I are thinking of moving away from here...if she recovers all right?"

Bairstow doesn't think he's heard right. "Moving? Moving where? Why would you move?"

"We've always wanted to live in California, did you know that? We settled here directly from my residency, and now it's time to move on."

"You mean...June agrees?"

Potter nods. "She says, 'If I want to go...'"

"But this is not the time," Bairstow protests. "You can't go now. It's premature to even think of it.."

"I know, I know. We'll wait a while. I think things will be different between June and me if we shove on, find new goals. I haven't been the greatest husband, Bairstow. Gone on weekends. It hasn't been great on June--you told me that. You were right. There are great bike races in California..."

"Jeff, it'll take June weeks to fully recover..."

"She might as well do it in the sunshine. Southern California should be great. They have surgeons and cobalt machines and radiation on the West Coast, too, you know."

Bairstow feels as if he's been assaulted. The breath leaves his body. "When do you plan to leave?"

"A month or two. No hurry, June needs time to recover like you said. I know that. I called San Diego this morning. See, I know a few people in the hospital out there. They need someone pretty soon."

"But June…"

"They have moving companies which come and pack your stuff so you don't have to lift a hand--June wouldn't have to do anything. They even find you a house and facilitate the entire business."

Bairstow turns slowly, shaking his head wearily. "I wish you well, Potter. Maybe I even envy you a little. Sometimes I've thought I'd like to leave this area, too, if I were able…but my roots are here, I'm afraid, for better or for worse."

Potter takes Bairstow's hand and shakes it. "Thanks, man. I'll always remember you with affection, you know that? I think you even helped me to grow up a little, but I'm not sure if you're aware of that. By the way, the committee came by the other day and asked me what I thought of you as head of service. I told them they'd never find anyone better if they ransacked the entire country. I hope you get the post."

Bairstow smiles fleetingly. "I'm afraid Miriam would die. She's been trying to get me to give up some of my hours."

"You'll never give them up, Bairstow. You're the best surgeon of all of us, and you have the most vitality, too. You're just tired. Thanks, by the way, for all you're doing for June. If anyone can get her well, I know you can. She knows that, too."

Bairstow stuffs his green operating room cap into his pocket and chuckles. "I'm just a country surgeon, Jeff."

"The hell you are, my friend."

June's post-operative course passes without event; she improves day by day. Soon she can sit up easily, then take a few halting steps.

Bairstow allots a few extra minutes from his rounds each day to sit beside her bed.

On the second day after surgery, when she was fully awake, Bairstow had pulled up his chair beside her bed and sat watching her face as her eyes opened. Her color had improved, he noted, and the nurses had brushed her hair. "You're looking much better," he said. "How do you feel?"

"As if I'm going to live. You were here frequently yesterday, weren't you. I remember your face as in a dream, but I know it was you."

"Yes, I was here several times."

She had looked up at him with effort. "Did Jeff tell you about the West Coast? He says he did."

"You're happy about it?"

She lay motionless on the bed for a moment or two, then moved her head almost imperceptibly. "It may be the beginning for the two of us. He's trying, Ben, really trying. Maybe that's all that counts. Do you understand about it?"

Bairstow had touched her hand on the blanket. "Only too well. I wish I didn't. But I admire Potter in many ways, I always have."

"He's already found a house, did you know, and has an appointment to the staff? They seemed to work fast when they discovered he wanted to go. Apparently they need a surgeon out there as soon as Jeff can get away."

Bairstow had nodded slowly, reluctantly. "I'll miss you, June."

"And I, you, my dear. You've been a friend...just when I needed one. I wish I'd known you forever, Ben. Maybe this will have to be enough--for now."

"To the future, then. You know I wish you and Potter well always."

"We'll meet again, Ben, I know it. You always say I'm clairvoyant."

The day finally arrives when Bairstow, feeling June has successfully completed her rehab and is well enough to travel, discharges her. The nurses place her in a wheelchair for her trip to the door of the hospital where Potter waits to take her home. Bairstow, still in his white hospital coat, stands beside her waiting for Potter to bring his car around to the entrance. "I've sent duplicates of all your tests to the surgeon in San Diego," he says. "I know the man, actually; his name is Hudson. I've talked to him and heard him lecture. You'll be in good hands when you get there."

June's hair is brushed back into a pony tail, tied with a ribbon, and the nurses have placed a sweater about her shoulders. It's a warm day outside, so she's comfortable enough. "Not in as good hands as yours," June says, smiling up at him. "It will never be the same, Ben."

He is silent for a moment, his hand on the back of her arm. "I'm afraid not much will be the same, June, but in many ways it may be better."

"Goodby then, dear friend. I'll say it now, while we have privacy. I will think of you always and wish you well."

"And I'll wait to hear of you. Write and I promise to answer."

"You can count on it."

Two months later Bairstow runs into Hudson at a meeting of the American College of Surgeons in Boston. The eminent surgeon has been asked to address regional physicians of the medical society at the Massachusetts General Hospital on techniques involving insertion of diagnostic dyes into a patient's blood stream. On the second day of the conference, Bairstow finds himself sitting at Hudson's table for lunch. Hudson slaps Bairstow on the back.

"Congratulations, Ben," he says. "They tell me you're chairman of surgery at Memorial. Potter told me. He's a terribly good man you sent out our way."

"How's his wife?" Bairstow asks. "June Potter? I understand you saw her a couple months ago."

"She's doing extremely well. Didn't Potter tell me that you're coming out our way soon? To that surgical conference at the end of the month? I understand you'll be conferring with our teams on staff mediation."

"I'm looking forward to it." Actually, he's spoken with June this very morning, and knows that she is almost well, that she'd lost her beautiful hair at the beginning of chemotherapy, but that it has grown back. "Actually, I'll be staying with the Potters."

"A stunning woman, Potter's wife," Hudson continues. "They entertained us at dinner a couple weeks ago, and all she did was pump me about you."

"I'm looking forward to seeing both of them."

"Well, look me up when you're there, Bairstow. Listen, have you heard the one about the surgeon who's shooting ducks with an internist? Well, the surgeon is sitting in the boat, aiming his gun, and the internist falls out..." Bairstow listens politely, but he's heard it 30 times already, and his mind is in San Diego, with a beautiful woman he knows.